Resuscitation

Handbook

An Essential Slide Collection of Resuscitation Techniques, based on the contents of this book, is available. The collection consists of numbered 35mm colour transparencies of each illustration in the book, and each section is accompanied by a slide index for easy reference. The material is presented in an attrative binder, which also contains a copy of the Handbook. Further information is available from:

Times Mirror International Publishers Limited
Lynton House
7–12 Tavistock Square
London WC1H 9LB
UK

Resuscitation
Handbook

SECOND EDITION

Peter J F Baskett BA MB BCh BAO FRCA

Consultant Anaesthetist
Frenchay Hospital and The Royal Infirmary,
Bristol, UK

With a contribution on paediatric resuscitation by

David A Zideman QHP(C) OStJ BSc (Hons) MB BS FRCA

M Mosby-Wolfe

London Baltimore Bogotá Boston Buenos Aires Caracas Carlsbad, CA Chicago Madrid Mexico City Milan Naples, FL
New York Philadelphia St. Louis Sydney Tokyo Toronto Wiesbaden

Publisher:	Fiona Foley
Project Manager:	Alan Burgess
Designer:	Mark Willey
Illustrator:	Marion Tasker
Production:	Susan Bishop
Indexer:	Anne McCarthy

Text set in Garamond; captions set in Gill.
Originated in Hong Kong by Mandarin Offset (HK) Ltd.
Printed in Hong Kong.
Produced by Mandarin Offset (HK) Ltd.

Cataloguing in Publication Data:
Catalogue records for this book are available from the British Library and the US Library of Congress.

ISBN 1-56375-620-X

For full details of all Times Mirror International Publishers Limited titles please write to:
Times Mirror International Publishers Limited
Lynton House
7–12 Tavistock Square
London WC1H 9LB
UK

PREFACE

The Second edition follows the same format and style as the first and is only slightly enlarged in size. However, much of the text has been re-written and many new and modified illustrations are included. The section on advanced airway management has now been extensively revised to take account of the increasing use of the laryngeal mask and the introduction of new airways and techniques. Active compression and decompression of the chest is described, being a new technique designed to improve cardiac output in resuscitation, Protocols and algorithms incorporate the 1992 European and UK Resuscitation Council Guidelines and those of the American Heart Association made in the same year. Recent modifications in trauma life support practice have been incorporated.

Finally, in response to popular demand, a new section on Paediatric Resuscitation has been included and is written by David Zideman to whom I am most grateful.

Peter J F Baskett *Bristol 1993*

ACKNOWLEDGEMENTS

I would like to thank my fellow members of the European Resuscitation Council, the Resuscitation Council UK and the Cardiopulmonary Resuscitation Committee of the World Federation of Societies of Anaesthesiologists, and my instructors from the American Heart Association's Advanced Cardiac Life Support Instructors Course and from the combined American College of Surgeons and Royal College of Surgeons Advanced Trauma Life Support Instructors Course, who have inspired me to write this manual.

I am also indebted to my colleagues, especially Marion Tasker, Alan Burgess and Mark Willey, at Gower Medical Publishing who have contributed substantially to the concept, illustrations, design and editing of this publication.

Finally, I would thank Jean Parr-Burman who has typed every word of the first edition and to Kathy Graham who typed all the revisions for the second edition. Both in their turn made my life possible.

For Simon, Lucy and Olivia

CONTENTS

Section I

INTRODUCTION

INTRODUCTION

THE CAUSES OF CARDIORESPIRATORY ARREST

Potentially reversible cardiorespiratory insufficiency and arrest is ultimately due to:

> **asphyxia**
> either caused by a non-respirable atmosphere airway obstruction
>
> or hypo-ventilation/apnoea
>
> or illness or injury which produces:
>
> **cardiocirculatory arrest**
> from a primary or secondary cause.

Each of these final pathways has a number of causes and precipitating factors (Figs 1.1–1.4). In the majority of patients the cause or causes will be obvious from the surrounding circumstances and a preliminary examination of the victim but, in some, more extensive assessment and investigation will be necessary.

All of these causes of cardiocirculatory arrest can lead to either ventricular fibrillation (VF), electro-mechanical dissociation (EMD) or asystole. Some of the causes predispose more frequently to one of these arrhythmias in particular. For instance, primary myocardial ischaemic disease gives rise to initial cardiac arrest more often in the form of ventricular fibrillation than in the form of asystole. Vagal stimulation generally results in asystole directly, and tension pneumothorax and cardiac tamponade frequently produces electromechanical dissociation. Asphyxial causes from unrespirable atmospheres, airway obstruction and apnoea normally produces asystole or electromechanical dissociation.

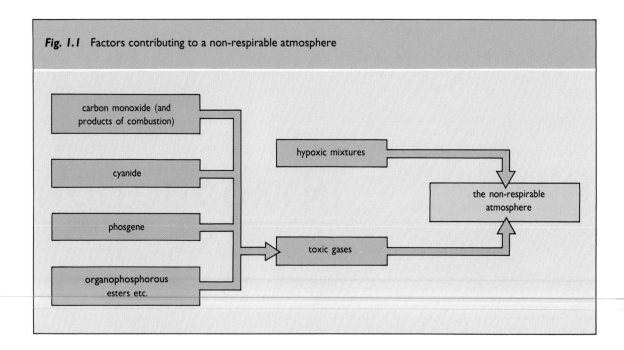

Fig. 1.1 Factors contributing to a non-respirable atmosphere

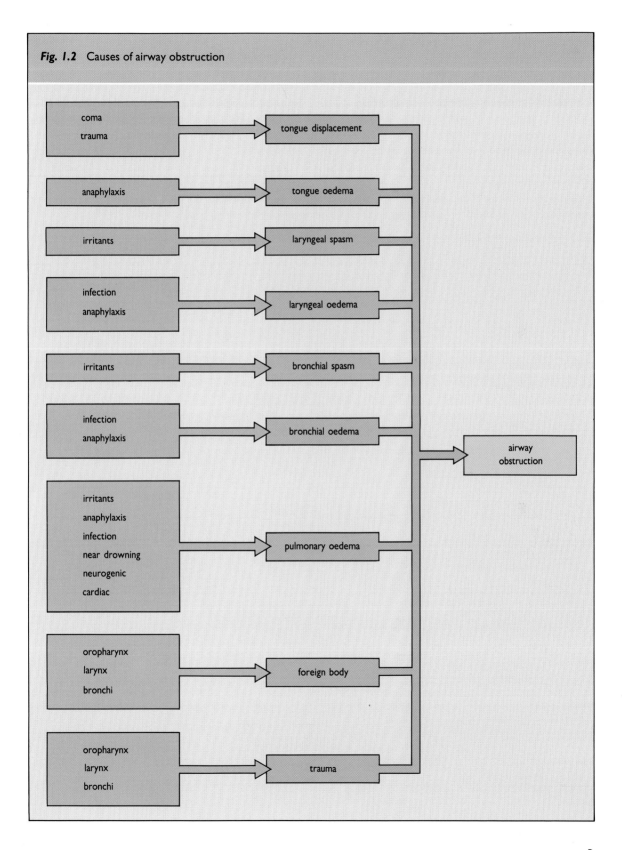

Fig. 1.2 Causes of airway obstruction

It should be remembered that all cases of ventricular fibrillation and electromechanical dissociation progress rapidly to asystole if left untreated.

Causes most susceptible to resuscitation

Although reports exist of survival from all the causes listed there are groups of patients in whom survival chances are substantial and those in whom outcome is almost universally poor.

Good results come from patients with ischaemic conduction defects which produce ventricular fibrilla-

tion initially. Prompt resuscitation and defibrillation can lead to hospital discharge with normal neurological function in between 35 and 50 per cent of cases. Encouraging survival patterns also occur with vagal and sympathetic excesses, certain poisons, electrocution, cardiac tamponade, hypothermia and acute electrolyte or acid-base disturbances, providing resuscitation and the appropriate treatment are implemented smartly (Fig. 1.5).

Poor results are associated with sepsis, the adult respiratory distress syndrome, massive cardiac infarction or failure, hepatorenal failure and hypovolaemia progressing to cardiac arrest (Fig. 1.6).

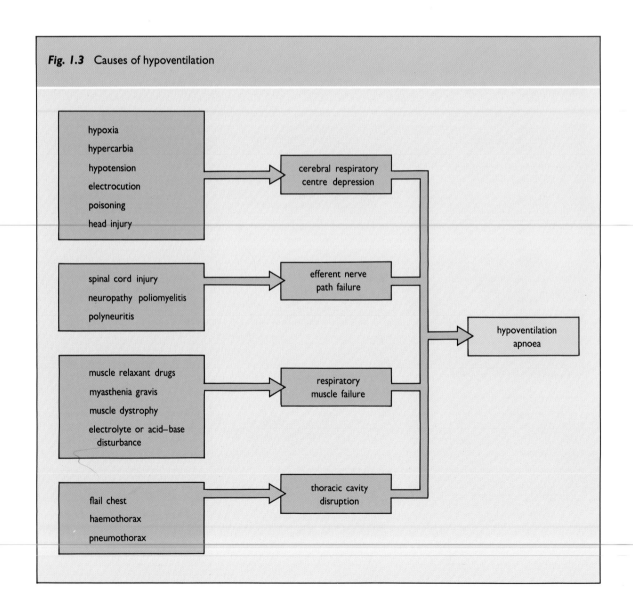

Fig. 1.3 Causes of hypoventilation

hypoxia
hypercarbia
hypotension
electrocution
poisoning
head injury

→ cerebral respiratory centre depression

spinal cord injury
neuropathy poliomyelitis
polyneuritis

→ efferent nerve path failure

muscle relaxant drugs
myasthenia gravis
muscle dystrophy
electrolyte or acid–base disturbance

→ respiratory muscle failure

flail chest
haemothorax
pneumothorax

→ thoracic cavity disruption

→ hypoventilation apnoea

The arrest of a previously healthy heart due to asphyxia frequently produces disastrous results. The healthy heart is a robust organ in comparison with the brain. Sufficient hypoxia to arrest a healthy heart is almost invariably associated with a greater or lesser degree of permanent cerebral damage. However, unbeknown to the rescuer, the heart may not have been completely healthy and may have arrested early before significant cerebral damage has occurred. Prompt resuscitation with restoration of an oxygenated circulation may prevent permanent neurological sequalae.

CEREBRAL SURVIVAL TIMES

Generally, cerebral neurones die after about 5 minutes of ischaemia. Certain factors however do influence these survival times for better or worse.

Factors which enhance survival times are hypothermia and certain drugs, such as barbiturates, benzodiazepines and calcium-blocking agents, if given fortuitously before the cardiac arrest occurs. All reduce cerebral oxygen requirements.

Children also may recover neurological function after periods of cardiac arrest which would cause

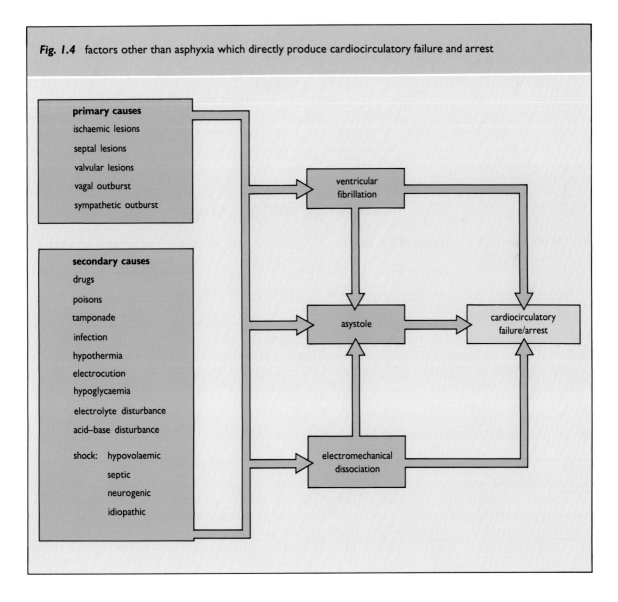

Fig. 1.4 factors other than asphyxia which directly produce cardiocirculatory failure and arrest

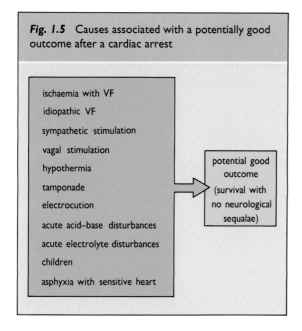

Fig. 1.5 Causes associated with a potentially good outcome after a cardiac arrest

ischaemia with VF

idiopathic VF

sympathetic stimulation

vagal stimulation

hypothermia

tamponade

electrocution

acute acid–base disturbances

acute electrolyte disturbances

children

asphyxia with sensitive heart

→ potential good outcome (survival with no neurological sequalae)

Fig. 1.6 Causes associated with a potentially bad outcome after a cardiac arrest

massive cardiac

infarction or failure

hepatic failure

prolonged asphyxia

hypovolaemia

sepsis

→ potentially bad outcome (death or permanent cerebral damage)

permanent damage in adults. The full extent of recovery may take several months to become apparent and is presumed to be due to recruitment and re-education of other neural tissue to take over the function of damaged areas.

PATIENTS WHO SHOULD NOT BE RESUSCITATED

Inappropriate resuscitation is morally unjustifiable and very poor medical practice. It denies the individual dignity in death — an event which ultimately overtakes us all. Because the resuscitation team has no time to review the patient's history in detail and because the (often junior) nurse with the patient cannot make a decision not to resuscitate on her own, each hospital should produce published guidelines for their policy of "Do Not Resuscitate". There can be no absolute rules, and every case must be judged on individual merits and the decision reviewed on an appropriate regular basis. It cannot be overemphasized that a decision not to resuscitate is absolutely compatible with continuing maximum nursing and therapeutic care.

The decision should be made in consultation with the patient, if appropriate or possible, or with family members and clearly recorded in the medical and nursing notes and duly signed, dated and reviewed regularly.

The decision will be based on a number of medical and social factors related to each individual's personal circumstances. Some of these factors are illustrated in Figure 1.7.

INFECTION HAZARDS IN RESUSCITATION

Infection may potentially occur after expired air resuscitation in either the rescuer or the victim.

Infection in the rescuer

Several organisms can, at least in theory, be transmitted by mouth to mouth contact (Fig. 1.8). However, in fact, the incidence of disease acquisition after resuscitation attempts is remarkably low. Isolated incidents of cutaneous tuberculosis, herpes labialis, meningococcal meningitis and shigellosis have been reported, but overall the risk is clearly extremely small.

The current principle fear of infection among would-be rescuers is the possibility of acquiring infection with the human immunodeficiency virus (HIV) from mouth to mouth contact with the victim. Although it is impossible to give an absolute guarantee that there is no risk, it has to be said that no case has been reported to date of the infection being acquired in this manner. Furthermore, a study of close non-sexual household contacts with casual exposure to saliva of HIV-positive individuals did not result in any spread of infection. Transmission of infection occurs much more readily with the Hepatitis B virus (HBV) and this, in practice, represents a much greater threat to rescuers.

It has been estimated that on average any individual, not acting as a health care professional, will be faced with a resuscitation opportunity no more than three or four times in a lifetime. Given that the possibility of acquiring an infection on any one of these occasions is minute, the rescuer should not be deterred from giving mouth to mouth resuscitation when the occasion arises. However, health care professionals are faced with many more occasions which require resuscitating victims of cardiorespiratory arrest and are dealing with a group of patients more likely to be suffering from an infection. The potential chances of transmission therefore are increased considerably in this group, and therefore it is recommended that simple ventilatory protection devices should be available for health care professionals as part of their portable equipment and at their place of work.

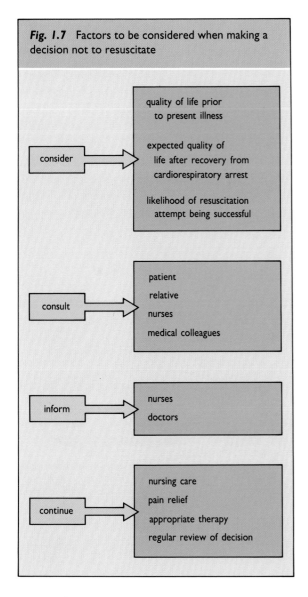

Fig. 1.7 Factors to be considered when making a decision not to resuscitate

consider → quality of life prior to present illness

expected quality of life after recovery from cardiorespiratory arrest

likelihood of resuscitation attempt being successful

consult → patient
relative
nurses
medical colleagues

inform → nurses
doctors

continue → nursing care
pain relief
appropriate therapy
regular review of decision

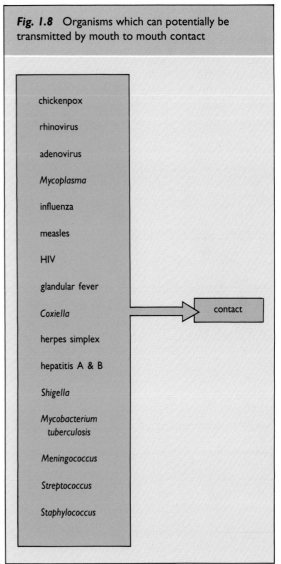

Fig. 1.8 Organisms which can potentially be transmitted by mouth to mouth contact

chickenpox

rhinovirus

adenovirus

Mycoplasma

influenza

measles

HIV

glandular fever

Coxiella   → contact

herpes simplex

hepatitis A & B

Shigella

Mycobacterium tuberculosis

Meningococcus

Streptococcus

Staphylococcus

Infection in the victim

Infection can also occur in the victim as a result of resuscitation attempts. Because the rescuer is usually a healthy individual it is most unlikely that an infection will be passed from rescuer to victim.

The commonest cause of infection in the victim is secondary respiratory tract infection arising after aspiration of foreign material – usually stomach contents. Infection may also occur (but surprisingly rarely) after hurried open chest cardiac compressions done without full aseptic precautions. Both infections are treated by supportive measures and definitive antibiotic therapy.

Simple resuscitation ventilatory devices

These devices are designed to enable expired air respiration (EAR) to be used whilst avoiding direct contact. In general there are two types of equipment: the anaesthetic face mask type and the tube/flange model which usually incorporates some form of oropharyngeal airway. Both types may be fitted with a one-way valve which diverts the victim's expired air away from the rescuer. An example of such devices is illustrated in Figure 1.9 and in Figure 2.50.

Generally it is easier to achieve an airtight seal with the patient's face with the mask type (e.g. the Laerdal Pocket Mask, the Seal/Vent Easy or the MTM Resuscitator). The tube/flange group (e.g. the Brook Airway, the Hi Tilt Airway, the Dual Aid, the Sussex Valve Airway and the Safar 'S' Airway) have the advantage of improving airway patency in some patients because of an oropharyngeal extension.

Protection devices made from a piece of simple, thin plastic film with a valvular orifice to cover the mouth and nose are available to the public for bystander resuscitation. They are very inexpensive and compact and are variously packed to resemble a cleansing tissue (Laerdal Resusciade) or to fit on a key ring (Ambu Life key, Fig. 1.10). The plastic film may tear around the valve in contact with teeth but by and large these appliances offer reasonable protection and reduce aesthetic worries of direct contact with patient's vomitus, saliva, sputum or blood.

DEFINITIONS OF DEATH

Clinical death

Clinical death is characterized by respiratory and cardiac arrest (Fig. 1.11). In certain patients the condition can be reversed by the prompt application of resuscitative measures.

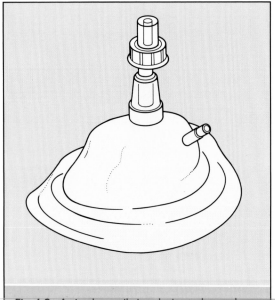

Fig. 1.9 A simple ventilation device to be used with EAR: the mask type

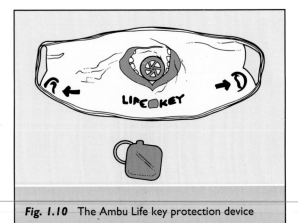

Fig. 1.10 The Ambu Life key protection device

Cerebral (cortical) death

Cerebral death is characterized by death of the cerebral hemispheres. The patient is deeply comatose but spontaneous breathing persists.

Brain stem death

Brain stem death is characterized by death of the brain stem and loss of all brainstem reflexes including spontaneous respiration. Brain stem death is generally accepted as "death" by most medical and legal authorities, even though the heart may continue to beat when supported by artificial ventilation. Organs may be removed, with permission, from brain stem dead donors whose heart continues to beat.

Brain death

Brain death is the death of all brain tissue — cerebrum, cerebellum, midbrain and brain stem. Spinal cord reflexes may however be present. Spontaneous respiration does not occur and organ donation is possible with permission.

Biological death

Clinical death is inevitably followed by biological death if no resuscitation is carried out. It comprises death and necrosis of all tissues starting with the brain, followed by the heart, kidneys, lung, liver, etc., and ending finally with the skin.

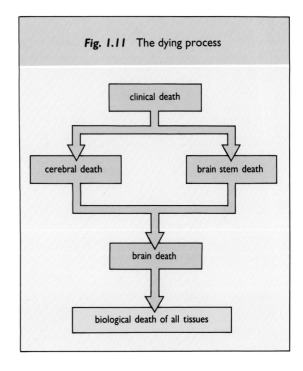

Fig. I.II The dying process

CARDIAC LIFE SUPPORT

LIFE SUPPORT IN RESUSCITATION

ASSESSMENT

Prior to beginning resuscitation the situation and the patient must be assessed. Ensure that a defibrilillator and advanced cardiac life support facilities are available or sent for.

> **Is the situation safe?**
> non-respirable atmosphere
> danger of electrocution
> danger from traffic
> danger from falling masonry
> The rescuer is obliged to make sure that he or she is in no personal danger: a second patient merely compounds the problem.

The unwitnessed collapse

In many instances, the collapse will not be witnessed by the rescuer who may have little or no idea of the cause or underlying disease. Assessment must therefore follow a methodical line to establish the precise nature of the problem, be it airway obstruction or respiratory or cardiocirculatory arrest. Only a very preliminary examination of the victim is required before starting resuscitation.

> **Two questions only need to be answered initially:**
> Is the patient unconscious?
> Does the patient have a deathlike appearance?
> (very pale, very grey or very blue)

If the victim fulfills both of these criteria then follow the Basic Life Support algorithm (Fig. 2.1) which is applicable to all cases of unwitnessed collapse.

The witnessed collapse

In some instances the collapse may be witnessed by the rescuer who may be able to decide the cause (e.g. drowning, head injury, choking, heart attack, etc).

Many patients who collapse due to an arrest from a primary cardiac cause do so from a sudden serious dysrhythmia. Prior to the event, respiratory function has been adequate and the blood in the vascular bed is well oxygenated. Their urgent need is for external chest compression to circulate the oxygenated blood to the brain. To accommodate this priority the algorithm may be modified in certain cases of suspected primary cardiac arrest (Fig. 2.2).

CLEARANCE AND MAINTENANCE OF THE AIRWAY USING BASIC LIFE SUPPORT TECHNIQUES

The Airway

An obstructed airway very commonly occurs in patients needing resuscitation. The commonest cause of obstruction in the supine position is the relaxed tongue falling back to obliterate the oropharynx posteriorly (Fig. 2.3).

Other common causes of airway obstruction are aspiration of regurgitated gastric contents and blood from the oro- or nasopharynx in maxillofacial injuries. Obstruction can also occur at laryngeal level from choking on a bolus of food or foreign bodies (particularly in children).

Classically the patient who is choking indicates his predicament by clasping his neck or pointing to his larynx with a finger.

Fig. 2.1 Algorithm for Basic Life Support in the unwitnessed collapse.

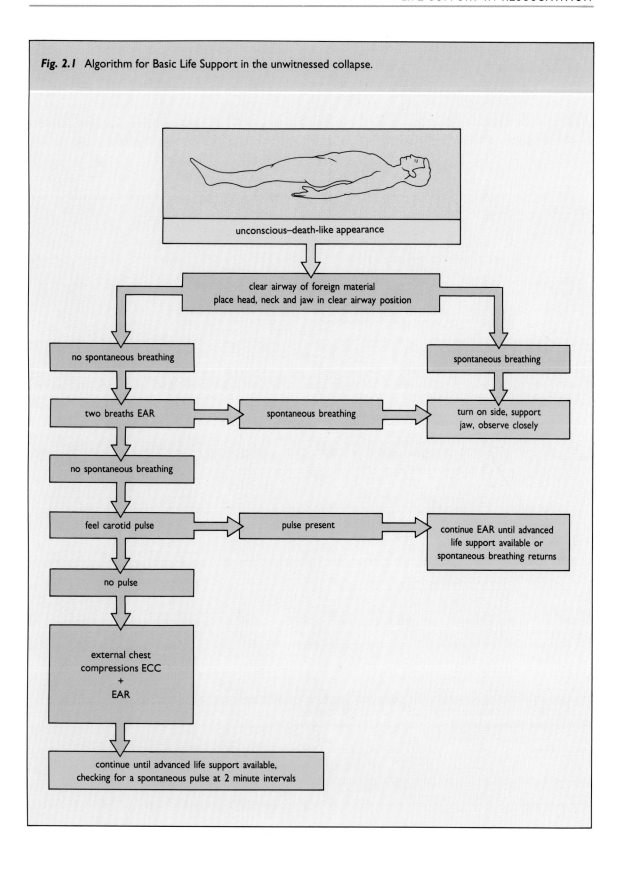

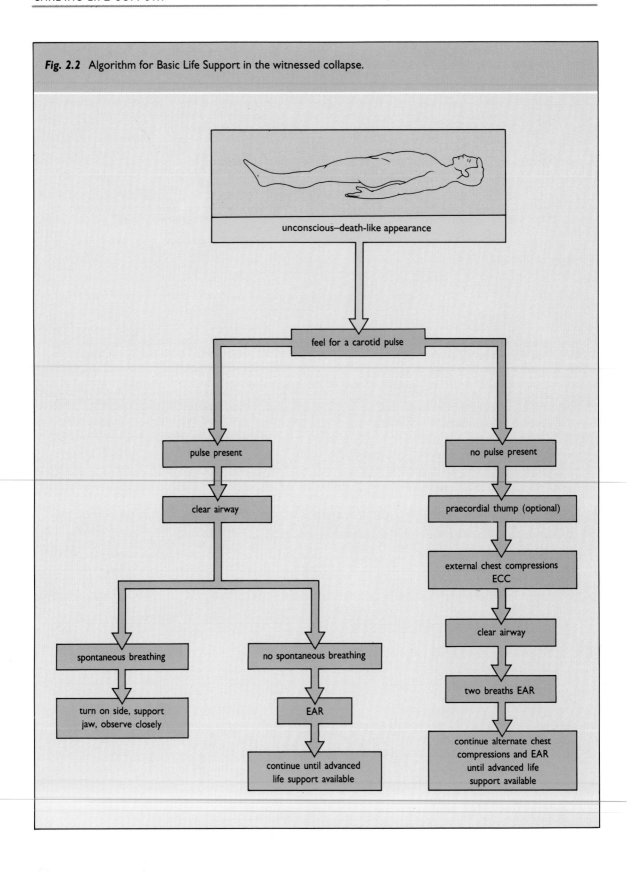

Fig. 2.2 Algorithm for Basic Life Support in the witnessed collapse.

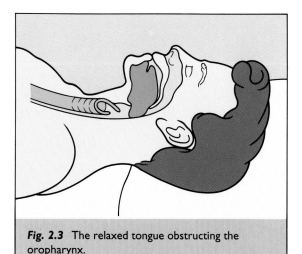

Fig. 2.3 The relaxed tongue obstructing the oropharynx.

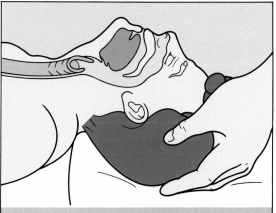

Fig. 2.4 Backward tilt of the head to open the airway.

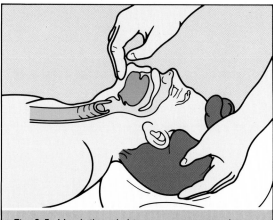

Fig. 2.5 Head tilt and chin support to open the airway.

The airway may be cleared and maintained by a number of manoeuvres which do not require equipment and therefore are included in Basic Life Support (BLS).

Positional Methods

Obstruction of the oropharynx by the tongue can be relieved by correct alignment of the head, neck and mandible, as described below. The combination of head tilt, jaw thrust and open mouth is known as the 'triple airway manoeuvre'.

Backward tilt of the head of the neck

In the majority of cases the obstruction by the tongue can be overcome by simple backward tilting of the head, which stretches the structures in the front of the neck and lifts the base of the tongue off the posterior pharyngeal wall (Fig. 2.4).

Technique
1   Ideally, the patient's head should be on a small pillow.
2   Tilt the head backwards; in the supine position this may be achieved by pushing the occiput or pressing on the forehead.

Great care should be taken with this manoeuvre in patients with suspected fractures of the cervical spine. Flexion and rotation of the neck are the most dangerous movements and extension of the head and neck should be minimized to that necessary to just establish an airway.

Chin support

The tongue is a muscle arising from the mandible and further relief of the obstruction may be provided by lifting the chin (Fig. 2.5).

Technique
1   Ideally, the patient's head should be on a small pillow.
2   Lift the chin: this pulls the tongue forward.

Jaw thrust

Even with head tilt, in some patients the tongue can only be pulled forward from the back of the pharynx by using the jaw thrust (Fig. 2.6).

Technique

1 Lift the mandible upwards and forwards with the index fingers placed just proximal to the angle.
2 Reach forward with the thumbs to depress the point of the chin to open the mouth slightly.

Recovery position

Once the airway has been cleared and established and adequate spontaneous respiration is assured then the patient should be turned into the lateral recovery position. There is some debate as to the best lateral position. Some prefer the lower leg to be flexed (Fig. 2.7), others prefer the upper leg to be flexed (Fig. 2.8). Either is suitable in many cases.

Technique

1 Turn the patient into the lateral recovery position, ensuring that the patient is "locked" in the lateral position and cannot roll back spontaneously into the supine position or forward into the prone position.
2 Maintain moderate head tilt by placing the patient's upper hand under his lower cheek.
3 Apply chin support or jaw thrust.
4 In the case of suspected spinal injury the head should not be turned in isolation but the entire patient should be "log rolled" into the lateral position, with an assistant holding the head, neck and chest in alignment (Fig. 2.9).

Clearance of the Airway Obstructed by Foreign Material

If the upper airway is obviously obstructed by foreign material in the hypopharynx, or if positive pressure ventilation attempts meet with resistance in spite of a clearly aligned airway, then the airway may be cleared by manual methods.

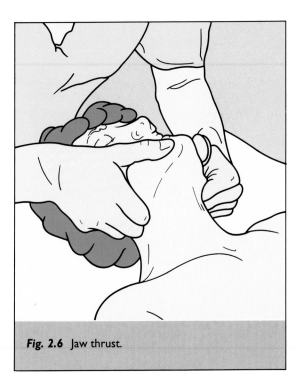

Fig. 2.6 Jaw thrust.

Finger sweeps

Finger sweeps are used to clear the airway in unconscious patients.

Technique — solid material

1 Force the mouth open, using the jaw thrust/chin depression method in the relaxed jaw (the Esmarch manoeuvre) or prise the mandible and maxilla apart anteriorly in the partly relaxed jaw (Fig. 2.10).
2 Sweep or hook the obstruction, preferably with fingers wrapped in a handkerchief or similar material.
3 The rescuer should beware of finger injury in sitting patients.

Technique — liquid material

1 Place the patient in the head down position.
2 Turn the head to one side.
3 Perform the manoeuvre as for solid material.

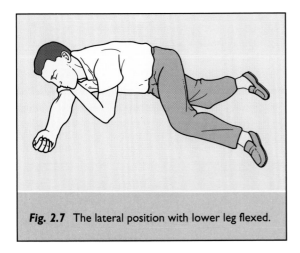

Fig. 2.7 The lateral position with lower leg flexed.

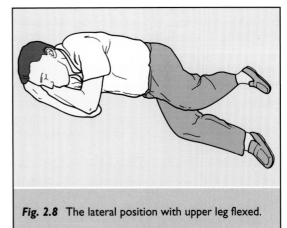

Fig. 2.8 The lateral position with upper leg flexed.

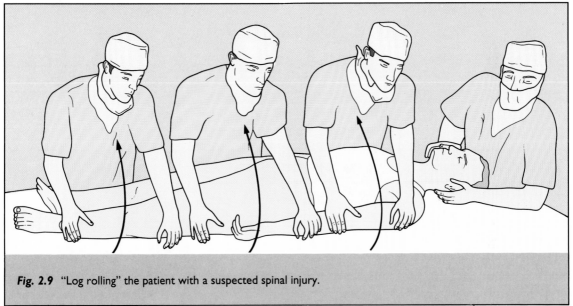

Fig. 2.9 "Log rolling" the patient with a suspected spinal injury.

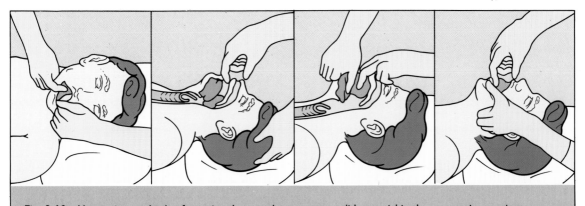

Fig. 2.10 Alternative methods of opening the mouth to remove solid material in the unconscious patient.

Back blows

In conscious patients with upper airway obstruction from foreign bodies, which is not relieved by coughing, the airway must be cleared by back blows. In adults the usual cause of such obstruction is a bolus of unchewed food — in children it can be a variety of objects.

Note: The technique of back blows is recommended by the World Federation of Anaesthesiologists, the Resuscitation Council (UK) and the European and Australian Resuscitation Councils. The American Heart Association recommends back blows in children but not in adults.

Technique

1 The patient ideally should be lying on his side, but the manoeuvre can also be performed with the patient sitting or standing and leaning forward (Fig. 2.11).
2 Children can be placed head down lying along the rescuer's thigh or arm (Fig. 2.12).
3 Give a series of four to six blows to the ▪▪▪▪▪ middle of the back during expiration, such that the high expiratory flow rate may expel the impacted material.

Abdominal thrusts (The Heimlich manoeuvre)

Abdominal thrusts may expel an impacted foreign body from the airway in conscious patients when back blows have failed.

Technique

1 Stand behind the victim, wrapping the arms around the patient just below the lower margin of the rib cage.
2 Clasp the hands tightly together and give a series of sharp upward thrusts, timed with expiration if discernible (Fig. 2.13).
3 Hopefully the increased expiratory flow rate will expel the offending obstruction. If it does not, be prepared for the victim to lose consciousness. If this occurs, attempt to remove the foreign body by finger sweeps.

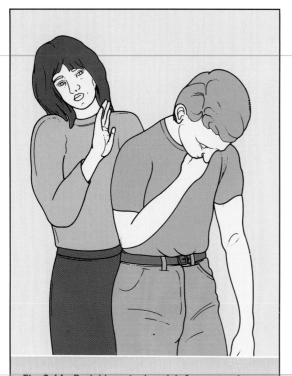

Fig. 2.11 Back blows in the adult for upper airway

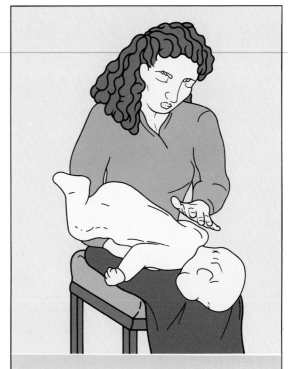

Fig. 2.12 Back blows in small children.

The Heimlich manoeuvre is not without danger. Visceral injury to the stomach, liver, spleen, aorta and diaphragm have been reported. The technique is not recommended in pregnancy, extreme obesity or infants and children.

CLEARANCE AND MAINTENANCE OF THE AIRWAY USING ADVANCED LIFE SUPPORT TECHNIQUES

If airway obstruction cannot be relieved by Basic Life Support measures, advanced measures using equipment will be required.

Foreign Body Clearance

Foreign material may be removed under direct vision in the unconscious patient using a laryngoscope, suction and forceps.

Technique

1 Align the head and neck in the optimal airway position.
2 Introduce the laryngoscope into the right hand corner of the mouth with the blade aiming towards the midline at laryngeal level.
3 Lift the handle of the laryngoscope upwards and forwards (towards the junction of the ceiling and the opposite wall) but do not on any account pull it backwards as this endangers the front teeth and also obscures the view of the hypopharynx (Fig. 2.14).
4 Using a Yankaeur design suction end, clear the liquid material by aspiration and pick out solid material under direct vision using Magill's offset forceps (Fig. 2.15).

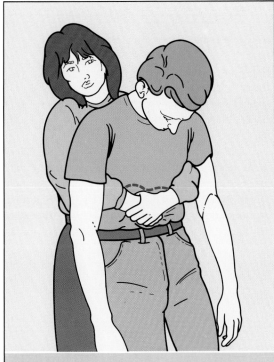

Fig. 2.13 Abdominal thrusts — the Heimlich manoeuvre.

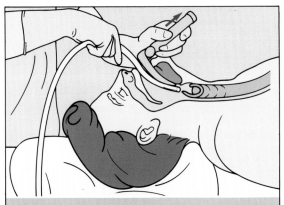

Fig. 2.14 Laryngoscopy and suction for clearing the airway of liquid material.

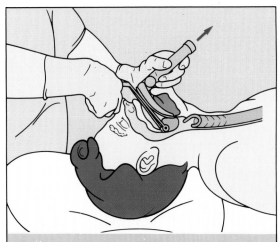

Fig. 2.15 Removal of solid foreign material using Magill's offset forceps.

Portable Suction Apparatus

Effective suction apparatus is a vital piece of equipment in resuscitation to clear the oropharynx of secretions, blood, regurgitated gastric contents and vomitus.

In hospitals a suction source is generally available in all patient areas and is supplied from a central vacuum unit or from a venturi device associated with a gas pipeline. Mains-powered electric units act as a back-up system.

Outside hospitals portable apparatus must be used. Several models are available and they fall broadly into two groups: (1) electric powered, and (2) hand- or foot-powered.

Electric-powered devices

These devices operate from rechargeable batteries. Some also offer additional mains (110 or 220V) or 12V power options to help with battery economy when such sources of power are available.

Points to be considered in selection of a suitable unit include:

- Performance: generation of adequate vacuum and flow rate to ensure easy aspiration of semi-solid tenacious material.
- Suitable fittings to attach Yankaeur suction ends, suction catheters or a suction booster device.
- A container for aspirated material of adequate size.
- Power source options of rechargeable battery, 12V, or mains supply.
- Size and weight in relation to portability.
- Ease of disassembly, cleaning and reassembly without potential error.
- Reliability in clinical use.
- Robust manufacture of suction unit, suction receptacle, carrying case and catches.

Examples of very effective devices include the Impact Portable Suction Unit (Fig. 2.16) and the Laerdal Portable Electric Suction Unit (Fig. 2.17).

Hand- or foot-powered devices

These devices have the advantage that they do not depend on an electric or mechanical source. Some models offer the option of conversion to a mechanical source of vacuum if one is available.

Foot-powered models (Fig. 2.18) leave the hands of the rescuer free for other tasks but may be difficult to operate in a moving ambulance or helicopter. Hand-powered models (Fig. 2.19) require both hands of the operator: one to power the device and the other to manipulate the suction end in the pharynx. The points to be considered in selection are very much the same as for portable electric suction units. Clearly hand-held units must be very lightweight.

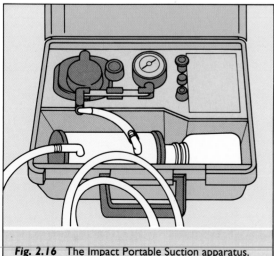

Fig. 2.16 The Impact Portable Suction apparatus.

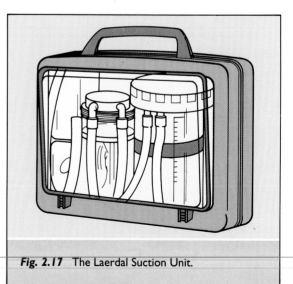

Fig. 2.17 The Laerdal Suction Unit.

Examples of very effective devices include the Ambu Foot or Hand Uni-Suction Pump (see Fig. 2.18) and the Vitalograph New Aspirator (see Fig. 2.19). The relatively small aspiration chamber of the Vitalograph New Aspirator is compensated for by an overflow arrangement (which may soil the operator's clothing unless care is taken!).

The suction booster

This device consists of a receptacle which is connected to the suction source by suction tubing and a wide-bore (15mm) tube for aspirating semi-solid vomitus. An effective sample is the Ambu Suction Booster (Fig. 2.20).

Airway Maintenance

Although a clear airway can generally be maintained without artificial aids on a short term basis, there are occasions when these are both helpful and necessary.Both the oropharyngeal and nasopharyngeal airways can be conveniently carried in the pocket.

The oropharyngeal (Guedel) airway

The oropharyngeal airway is a useful aid in controlling backward displacement of the tongue in the unconscious victim reducing the need for prolonged application of jaw thrust.

Technique

I Introduce the airway into the mouth in the inverted position and rotate it through 180° as it passes beneath the palate and into the oropharynx (Fig. 2.21).

In patients with active glossopharyngeal and laryngeal reflexes the oropharyngeal airway may provoke retching, vomiting, aspiration or laryngeal spasm. Remove the airway at the first sign of these events.

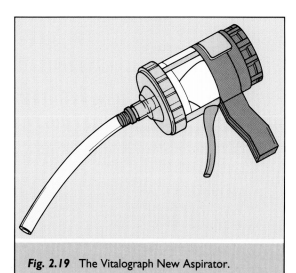

Fig. 2.19 The Vitalograph New Aspirator.

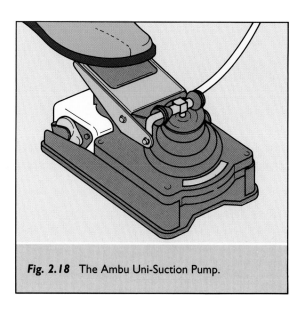

Fig. 2.18 The Ambu Uni-Suction Pump.

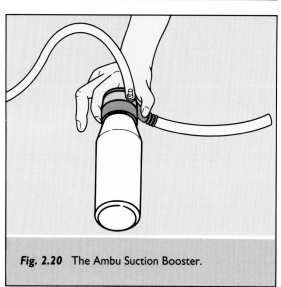

Fig. 2.20 The Ambu Suction Booster.

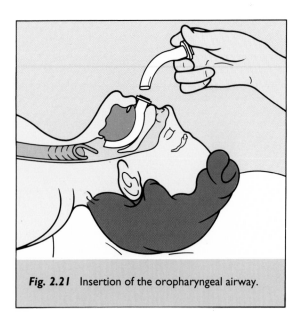

Fig. 2.21 Insertion of the oropharyngeal airway.

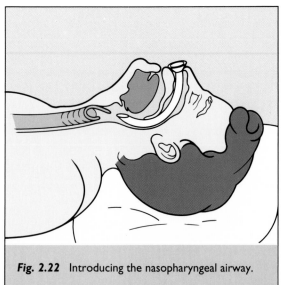

Fig. 2.22 Introducing the nasopharyngeal airway.

The nasopharyngeal airway

The nasopharyngeal airway (Fig. 2.22) is introduced via either nostril and passes through the nasopharynx so that the tip is just above the laryngeal opening. It is of particular value in maxillofacial injuries, patients with clenched jaws and on occasions when the oropharyngeal airway is rejected or provokes retching or laryngeal spasm. The airway should be made of soft material to minimise nasal injury.

Technique

1 The airway must be well lubricated before use.

2 In non-urgent use the nose should be sprayed with a solution of cocaine, 5–10% with adrenaline, to minimize haemorrhage from the nasal mucous membrane, but there is not time to do this in an emergency situation and so this preparation must be omitted.

3 A 6.0 or 6.5mm diameter airway is suitable for adults and should be introduced gently into the right nostril first. If nasal obstruction is encountered withdraw the airway and use the left nostril.

4 Suction should be on hand to control any nasal bleeding (which however is rarely a serious problem if care is taken).

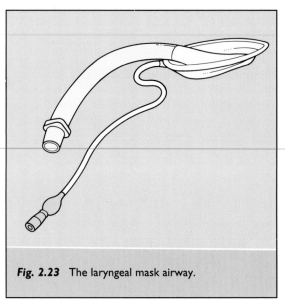

Fig. 2.23 The laryngeal mask airway.

The laryngeal mask airway

This device is a new design of oral airway, consisting of a tube with an elliptical cuff fitted at the distal end which inflates posteriorly in the hypopharynx around the posterior perimeter of the larynx. The tube is introduced so that it abuts on to the laryngeal isthmus and the cuff inflated to form an airtight seal. The potential advantage of the laryngeal mask airway is that it can provide a clear and secure airway without the need for the skill required for laryngoscopy and endotracheal intubation.

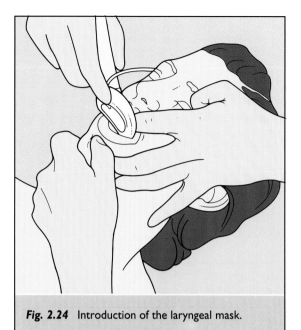

Fig. 2.24 Introduction of the laryngeal mask.

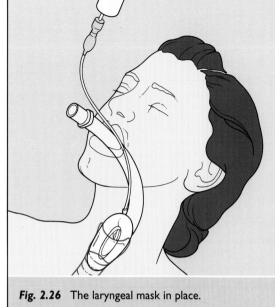

Fig. 2.26 The laryngeal mask in place.

Fig. 2.25 Sizing and inflation volumes for the laryngeal mask

Patient	Weight	Size	Cuff Volume
Neonates/infants	up to 6.5kg	1	2–4ml
Infants/children	6.5–15kg	2	10ml
Children	15–30kg	2.5	15ml
Small adults/children	30–50kg	3	20ml
Normal and large adults	>50kg	4	30ml

Technique

1 Deflate the cuff completely so that it forms a flat oval disc without any wrinkles (Fig. 2.23).
2 Lubricate the back of the mask and the posterior rim of the cuff thoroughly just before use. Do not lubricate the anterior aspect of the mask.
3 Align the head and neck in the clear airway position so that the neck is moderately ▪▪▪▪▪ flexed and the head is extended at the atlanto-occipital joint by occipital downward pressure with the non-dominant hand. Have an assistant open the mouth by depressing the chin.
4 Holding the tube like a pen, introduce the laryngeal mask into the mouth with the aperture facing caudally. Advance the tip with steady application upwards against the surface of the hard and soft palates, observing that the distal tip remains flat during insertion until it reaches the posterior pharyngeal wall (Fig. 2.24).
5 Maintaining the mask in position move the operating hand to the proximal end of the tube and press the mask into position so that the tip locates in the base of the hypopharynx. At this point resistance is felt and the airway is correctly placed. The black line on the tube should be aligned with the nasal septum.
6 Inflate the cuff with the recommended volume of air (Fig. 2.25). Note that the tube rises out of the mouth slightly (1–2cm) and that the larynx is pushed anteriorly as the mask finds its correct position (Fig. 2.26).▪▪▪▪▪

•••••7 Confirm that the airway is clear in the spontaneously breathing patient by listening for breath sounds at the proximal end of the tube.

8 In apnoeic patients correct placement is confirmed by attempting positive pressure ventilation and assessing inflation pressure, chest movement, lung auscultation and leakage around the cuff.

9 Insert a gauze or plastic bite block beside the tube and tie or tape the airway in place ensuring that the black line on the tube is aligned with the nasal septum.

Provided that the correct technique and indications for insertion are followed few problems occur with the use of the laryngeal mask.

Difficulties which may be experienced include:

- Rejection, coughing, straining and laryngeal spasm in patients who are not profoundly unconscious.
- Incorrect placement due to folding of the mask tip during insertion (Fig. 2.27). Withdraw the tube and start again making sure the cuff is fully deflated.
- Airway obstruction due to downfolding of the epiglottis (Fig. 2.28). Withdraw the tube, deflate the cuff fully and ensure that the mask is applied firmly to the surface of the palate during insertion.
- Airway obstruction due to rotation of the mask. Always ensure that the black line on the tube is aligned with the nasal septum. Deflate the cuff, reposition correctly and re-inflate.
- Persistent leakage around the cuff during positive pressure ventilation may be due to incorrect sizing, inadequate cuff inflation, excessive inflation pressure or poor compliance of the patient's lungs.
- Inflation pressures should not exceed 20cm H2O. In the vast majority of patients adequate ventilation can be achieved below this inflation pressure with careful attention to technique.

With experience it is now clear that the laryngeal mask has a very useful role in resuscitation. The technique can easily be taught in a few hours to paramedics, nurses and doctors not experienced with endotracheal intubation on a regular basis. While not providing absolute protection against aspiration in 100 per cent of cases, the laryngeal mask offers considerably greater security compared with other oral or nasal airways except the endotracheal tube. Tracheal intubation requires extensive training and regular practice to maintain the skill compared

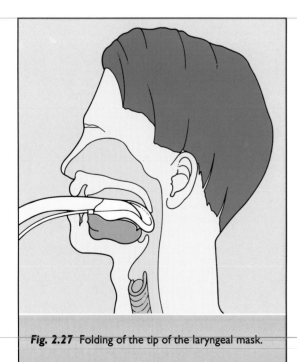

Fig. 2.27 Folding of the tip of the laryngeal mask.

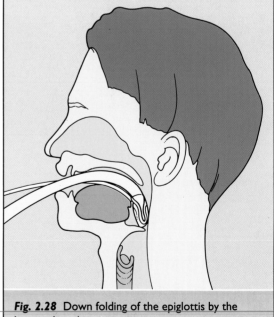

Fig. 2.28 Down folding of the epiglottis by the laryngeal mask.

with the laryngeal mask. It is likely that the laryngeal mask will become the initial airway management of choice in resuscitation for all but experienced tracheal intubationists.

The Pharyngo Tracheal Lumen Airway

The Pharyngo Tracheal Lumen Airway (PTLA) (Fig. 2.29) has been introduced in the United States largely as a replacement for the Oesophageal Obturator Airway and the Oesophageal Gastric Tube Airway which were waning in popularity. The device, which is passed blindly through the mouth, consists of two tubes. The longer tube has a distal cuff. The shorter tube, which extends just beyond a larger proximal cuff, is designed to be located in the pharynx. Normally, the longer tube passes into the oesophagus and its cuff is inflated to restrain regurgitated gastric contents from entering the airway. The proximal pharyngeal cuff is blown up to obliterate the hypopharynx and serves to tamponate bleeding points in this area. Inflation through the short tube will ventilate the lungs through the larynx. Alternatively, if the long tube enters the trachea the device simply acts as an endotracheal tube. The short tube then acts as a guidepath for a separate gastric tube to remove stomach contents.

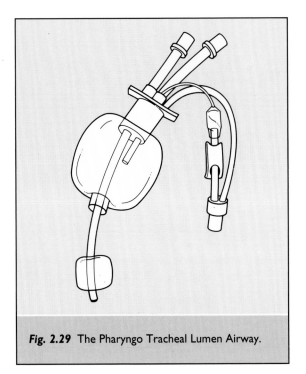

Fig. 2.29 The Pharyngo Tracheal Lumen Airway.

Technique

1 Lubricate both tubes and cuffs.
2 Align the head and neck in the clear airway position with the neck moderately flexed and the head extended at the atlanto-occipital joint by occipital downward pressure with the non-dominant hand.
3 An assistant should open the mouth by depressing the chin. Introduce first the longer tube into the mouth following the line of the hard and soft palates. As the shortest tube follows it will come to rest in the hypopharynx and the long tube will enter the oesophagus or trachea.
4 Inflate both cuffs simultaneously with 100ml of air through the common inflation port which incorporates a one way valve.
5 Ascertain if the long tube has entered the oesophagus or trachea by ventilating through it. If it has entered the trachea breath sounds will be heard and chest expansion on inspiration will occur. Ventilation will be as through an endotracheal tube and the short tube will serve as a drainage route for gastric contents. A gastric tube may be passed through the short tube to deflate the stomach.
6 If the long tube has entered the oesophagus (which is usual) breath sounds will be heard through the short tube which is thus the correct route for inflation.

The device is bulky and may be difficult to introduce in certain patients.
Excessive force may cause further damage to soft tissues and create a false passage in patients with intra-oral or pharyngeal injuries.
Disaster may occur if intermittent positive pressure is applied inadvertently to the long tube placed in the oesophagus or to the pharyngeal tube when the long tube has entered the trachea.

Overall, the laryngeal mask offers a better alternative than the PTLA because of its inherent simplicity and ease of insertion and absence of confusion in relation to the correct port for inflation.

The oesophageal tracheal Combitube airway

The Combitube is a double lumen tube which is designed to be passed blindly through the mouth. The patient can be ventilated whether the tube enters the trachea or the oesophagus.

The "tracheal" channel has an open distal end and the "oesophageal" channel has a blind distal end with openings at pharyngeal level. There is a cuff (10–15ml) placed distally and a large volume cuff (100ml) placed at hypopharyngeal level to seal off the nose and mouth.

If the tube enters the oesophagus ventilation can occur through the oesophageal channel via the pharyngeal holes and the laryngeal opening (Fig. 2.30).

If the tube enters the trachea ventilation of the lungs will not be possible via the oesophageal channel. Gastric inflation will occur through the pharyngeal holes. Ventilation of the lungs should be performed using the "tracheal" channel (Fig. 2.31).

There have been several reports of the successful use of the Combitube in situations when endotracheal intubation was not possible and during CPR. It is likely to find a useful place as a secure airway alternative.

Tracheal intubation

Tracheal intubation provides a reliable, clear and secure airway through which effective, positive pressure ventilation can be readily applied. It should be performed as soon as a skilled person is available in all cases of cardiorespiratory arrest lasting more than 2–3 minutes. Once the tube is in place with the cuff inflated the patient can be ventilated reliably without a leak and without the danger of inflating the oesophagus and stomach. Any regurgitated stomach contents will be safely contained in the pharynx and will not contaminate the respiratory tract.

The only drawback to the technique is that it does require considerable training and practice which takes some time to acquire. Initial training can take place on a manikin but real expertise only comes with practise on patients.

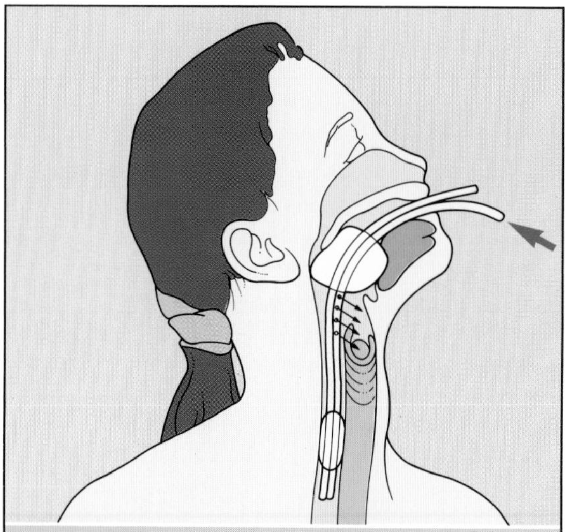

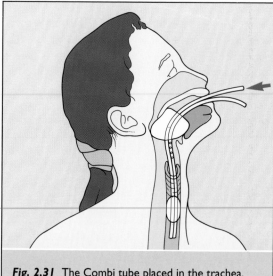

Fig. 2.31 The Combi tube placed in the trachea.

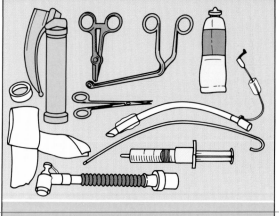

Fig. 2.32 The equipment needed for endotracheal

Fig. 2.30 The Combi tube placed in the oesophagus.

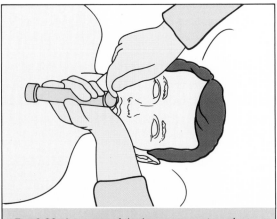

Fig. 2.33 Insertion of the laryngoscope into the mouth and hypopharynx.

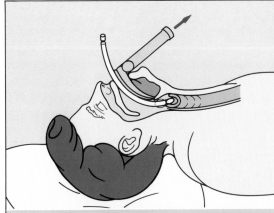

Fig. 2.34 Endotracheal intubation using a curved bladed laryngoscope.

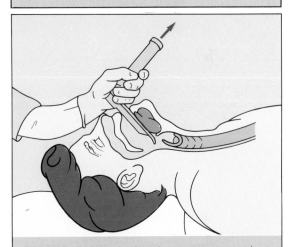

Fig. 2.35 Endotracheal intubation using a straight bladed laryngoscope.

Equipment for tracheal intubation using direct laryngoscopy

The equipment required for tracheal intubation is shown in Figure 2.32. This includes: a laryngoscope with appropriate size blades; a selection of oral and nasal endotracheal tubes of varying diameters and cut to the correct length with connectors to fit the ventilating apparatus; a syringe to inflate the cuff; a clamp for the cuff; a flexible stylet; lubricating jelly; Magill's forceps; a tape or bandage to secure the tube in place; and scissors.

Orotracheal intubation - under direct vision using laryngoscopy

Technique

1 Check that all the equipment is available and works, including tubes of correct length and diameter and batteries and bulb in laryngoscope.
2 Place patient in the supine position with the head on a low pillow.
3 Extend the head on the neck by pushing the occiput caudally.
4 With the left hand, insert the laryngoscope blade into the right hand corner of the mouth, ensuring that the lower lip is not caught between the blade and the lower teeth (Fig. 2.33). ▪▪▪▪▪

▪▪▪▪5 Advance the laryngoscope blade tip, aiming for the larynx in the midline, displacing the tongue towards the left side of the mouth.
6 Lifting the laryngoscope handle upwards and forwards (towards the junction of the ceiling and the opposite wall), slide the tip of the curved bladed laryngoscope between the base of the tongue and the root of the epiglottis, maintaining head tilt with occipital pressure with the right hand (Fig. 2.34). Note: If a straight bladed laryngoscope is used the tip of the blade should be placed beneath the epiglottis (Fig. 2.35). ▪▪▪▪▪▪

• • • • • Do not lean the laryngoscope blade on the upper teeth.

7 Visualize the larynx, adjusting the position of the tip of the blade for the best view (Fig. 2.36). Cricoid pressure may be helpful in bringing the larynx into line and reduces the possibility of gastric regurgitation.

8 Insert the lubricated endotracheal tube through the right hand corner of the patient's mouth and pass it between the vocal cords under direct vision. Rotate the tube if necessary for ease of insertion.

9 If a stylet is used it should be well lubricated with jelly and passed through the tube so that about 1cm protrudes at the distal end. Lock the stylet in this position by bending it over the tube connection at the proximal end. Under direct vision pass the stylet between the vocal cords and "railroad" the tube to follow the stylet into the trachea, rotating it gently if necessary. Once the tube is in the trachea the stylet should be removed by an assistant.

10 The tube should be advanced so that the cuff lies below the vocal cords.

11 The cuff is inflated through the pilot tube with air (or water under certain circumstances of variable atmospheric pressure) as continuous positive pressure ventilation is applied through the tube lumen using a self-inflating bag or anaesthetic circuit. A seal between the cuff and the trachea is signalled by the absence of an audible leak. If this does not occur after 10-15cm of air has been introduced into the cuff, check under direct vision that the tube is not placed in the oesophagus. Finally check that the tube is correctly placed by listening for breath sounds over both lung upper lobes and observe bilateral inspiratory and expiratory movements.

12 Secure the tube in place using adhesive tape or bandage. The entire procedure should not take more than 45 seconds in the apnoeic patient. If the attempt has failed after this time, remove the laryngoscope and tube and ventilate for 1–2 minutes with oxygen before trying again.

Nasotracheal intubation

Nasotracheal intubation (Fig. 2.37) is generally not used in the majority of patients with cardiorespiratory arrest because it is more difficult for most operators to carry out and because it carries with it the potential danger of nasal haemorrhage and infection with organisms carried from the nose into the trachea. Its use in the emergency situation should be reserved for occasions when orotracheal intubation is impossible, for example certain maxillofacial injuries and abnormal anatomical configurations such as ankylosing spondylitis.

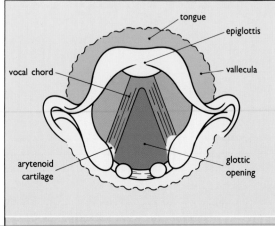

Fig. 2.36 The larynx viewed through a laryngoscope.

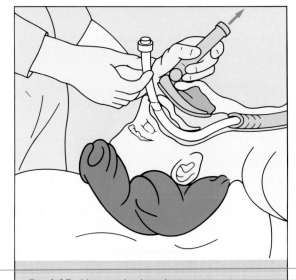

Fig. 2.37 Nasotracheal intubation.

The nasotracheal tube can be introduced blindly or placed between the vocal cords under direct vision.

> ### Technique
> 1 Place the patient in the supine position with the head on a pillow and with the head and neck aligned in the clear airway position by pressure on the occiput.
> 2 Attempt to introduce the well-lubricated nasotracheal tube through the right nostril (the nasal cavity runs more or less straight backwards). If significant resistance is met remove the tube and try the left nostril.
> 3 Pass the tube through the nasopharynx and steer it through the glottis into the trachea, with an assistant manipulating the larynx.
> 4 If resistance is met, or the tube passes into the oesophagus, introduce the laryngoscope to view the larynx in the same manner as for orotracheal intubation. Again attempt to steer the tip of the tube between the cords under direct vision, manipulating the tip of the laryngoscope blade, with an assistant manoeuvring the larynx.
> 5 If intubation is not possible, use Magill's offset forceps to grasp the tube in the nasopharynx one inch from the distal end and steer it through the glottis, with an assistant providing a gentle forward push on the tube at the nasal end.
> 6 If the tube appears to pass between the vocal cords but impinges anteriorly, it may be dislodged by rotation or by slight flexion of the head on the neck with continued downward pressure.
> 7 Once the tube is in place the cuff should be inflated and the correct position checked. It should be secured in place following a similar routine as for orotracheal intubation.

Alternative Methods Of Tracheal Intubation

A number of alternative methods of intubation have been devised. Some of these have been designed primarily to overcome problems in certain patients who have anatomical abnormalities which render intubation using direct laryngoscopy either difficult or impossible. Other techniques have been devised

to be simpler and require less manual dexterity and therefore to be more easily taught to paramedics, nurses, and non-specialist physicians. In general, however, they lack the high reliability of the direct laryngoscopy technique and they also require considerable practice.

Digital orotracheal intubation

With practise the majority of deeply comatose patients can be intubated by this method (Fig. 2.38) as long as the operator's fingers are long enough.

> ### Technique
> 1 The tube should be lubricated and fitted with a stylet curved to form a "J" shape.
> 2 Standing by the side of the patient, introduce the index and middle fingers into the corner of the mouth, depressing the tongue forwards until the epiglottis is reached and pulled forwards with the tongue.
> 3 Pass the tube into the mouth along a path between the two fingers towards the epiglottis and manoeuvre it just behind the epiglottis into the laryngeal opening.
> 4 Withdraw the stylet, check the tube position, inflate the cuff and secure the tube.

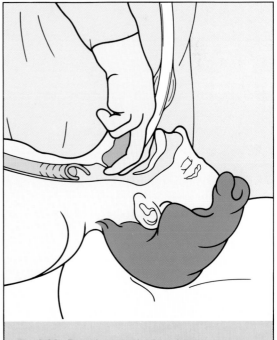

Fig. 2.38 Digital orotracheal intubation.

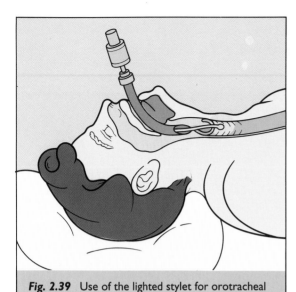

Fig. 2.39 Use of the lighted stylet for orotracheal intubation.

Orotracheal intubation using transillumination

In this technique (Fig. 2.39) a lighted stylet (light-stick) is passed through the lumen of the tube so that the lighted end just emerges from the distal end of the tube. The stylet is again bent so that the tube forms a "J" shape.

Technique

1 The technique of introduction of the tube into the mouth is similar to the digital method.

2 As the distal end of the tube reaches the back of the tongue, the light source illuminates the hypopharynx anteriorly. If the tube is advanced correctly into the trachea the intensity of the transillumination increases and is seen in the midline.

3 If the tube passes into the oesophagus, the transillumination is reduced. Transillumination to one side of the midline indicates incorrect positioning in the piriform fossa.

Fibreoptic laryngoscopic intubation

This technique (Fig. 2.40) is not appropriate for the emergency situation or the apnoeic patient except in very expert hands as it is much more time consuming than the other methods. It requires considerable practise to become reliably competent and is reserved for the "difficult intubation" not possible by other techniques.

Technique

1 Prepare the conscious patient by intravenous sedation with a small dose of benzodiazepine (e.g. Diazemuls 10mg or midazolam 5mg). Topical anaesthesia with 3–4ml of lignocaine 4% can be applied to the larynx using the transcricoid injection technique.

2 Prepare the nasal passages by spraying with a mixture of 10% cocaine and adrenaline to shrink the mucous membranes and reduce the chance of bleeding (which obscures the view through the laryngoscope).

3 Lubricate the tube and the flexible fibreoptic laryngoscope and introduce them through the nostril into the nasopharynx.

4 Advance the fibreoptic laryngoscope until the epiglottis and vocal cords come into view and then pass the tip through the larynx into the trachea.

5 Confirm the position of the laryngoscope by a view of the tracheal rings.

6 "Railroad" the tube itself over the fibreoptic laryngoscope into the trachea, inflate the cuff and secure the tube in the usual way.

Detection Of Correct Tracheal Tube Placement

Reliable confirmation of correct placement of the tracheal tube is vital if disaster with serious medico-legal consequences is to be avoided. Several methods are available.

Clinical Techniques

1 Visualize tube passing through vocal cords by direct laryngoscopy.

2 Insert finger alongside tube to feel it passing through the larynx.

3 Apply positive pressure ventilation with the cuff fully inflated and note:
  • absence of leak around cuff.
  • breath sounds heard in both axillae.
  • normal bilateral chest expansion with inflation.
  • absence of sounds in the epigastric area.

However, these checks have not proved reliable in 100 per cent of cases and so may be amplified by other methods.

Transillumination

A lighted stylet is passed through the tracheal tube. Correct placement in the trachea is confirmed by bright transillumination. Only a dull glow is seen if the tube is in the oesophagus. This method is not 100 per cent reliable and depends on background lighting and observer variations.

Fibreoptic Inspection

A fibreoptic bronchoscope or laryngoscope is passed through the lumen of the tracheal tube and correct placement is confirmed by the sight of the tracheal rings and carina. This is the most reliable method.

Carbon Dioxide Detection

Carbon dioxide emerging during expiration can be detected using a capnograph or an inexpensive CO_2 colourimetric detector. It should be noted that this method is unreliable in cardiac arrest with inadequate tissue perfusion since CO_2 is not being transported from the tissues to the lungs. End tidal CO_2 values do provide a useful indicator of the efficacy of CPR and may give some prediction of outcome. Values greater than 2kPa carry a good prognosis and less than 1.3kPa indicate a poor prognosis.

Oesophageal Detector

This is a simple inexpensive and reliable device. A 50ml syringe with a central nozzle is attached through a 20cm length of catheter mount corrugated tubing to a 15mm adaptor applied to the tracheal tube (Fig. 2.41). If the tracheal tube is correctly placed, air is easily aspirated. Resistance to aspiration indicates that the tube is in the oesophagus.

Cricothyrotomy

In a very small proportion of cases endotracheal intubation will prove impossible or inappropriate due to extensive maxillofacial injury or severe anatomical abnormality. In such patients cricothyrotomy may be the only method of establishing a clear airway. Cricothyrotomy is simpler to perform than tracheostomy which is fraught with difficulties and hazards in the emergency situation.

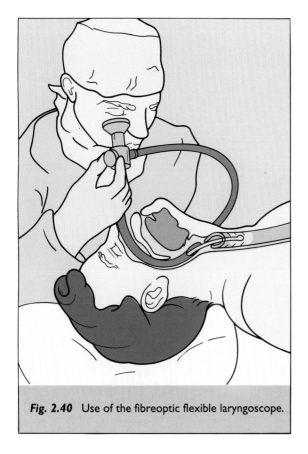

Fig. 2.40 Use of the fibreoptic flexible laryngoscope.

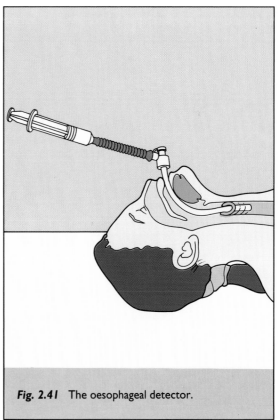

Fig. 2.41 The oesophageal detector.

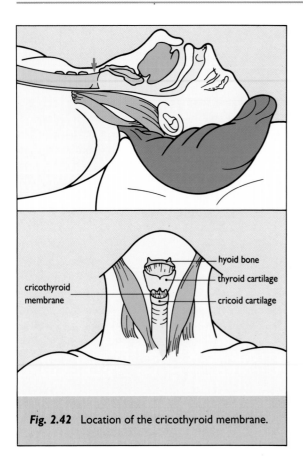

Fig. 2.42 Location of the cricothyroid membrane.

Technique

1 Place the patient in the supine position with the head fully extended on the neck.
2 Identify the cricothyroid membrane by palpation just below the thyroid cartilage (Fig. 2.42).
3 Make a 2–3cm skin incision with a scalpel and identify the cricothyroid membrane and incise it sufficiently to accommodate a 6.0mm tube in adults.
4 Pass a 6.0mm endotracheal or tracheostomy tube with connector through the incision under direct vision into the trachea and secure the tube in place (Fig. 2.43).

"Blind cricothyrotomy"

Purpose designed cricothyrotomy sets have been produced, for example the Portex Minitrach and the Nu-Trach. With each device a skin incision is first made with a scalpel over the cricothyroid membrane.

■ **THE PORTEX MINITRACH** (Fig. 2.44) consists of a bougie which is introduced through a small incision made in the skin and the membrane. Once the bougie is located in the trachea a tracheal tube is

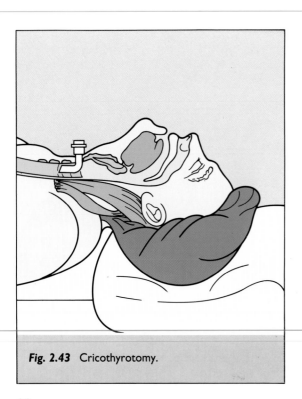

Fig. 2.43 Cricothyrotomy.

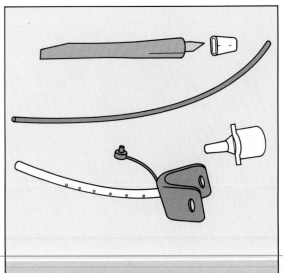

Fig. 2.44 The Portex Minitrach.

"railroaded" over it and the bougie withdrawn. Tubes of increasing size should be used as dilators, starting with the 4.0mm provided until a tube of 6.0–6.5mm is finally inserted. Practise is needed for expertise: it can be difficult to trace and locate the scalpel incision made in the membrane with the bougie by palpation only, especially in the gasping patient. The skin and membrane can be transfixed together by two needles placed laterally to the proposed incision through the cricothyroid membrane, to overcome this problem. An assistant is required to hold the larynx steady throughout the procedure. Bleeding can also present problems on occasion, particularly in the congested asphyxiating patient.

■ **THE NU-TRACH** consists of a patent trochar system with expandible diameter which pierces the membrane through a skin incision. A series of dilators of increasing sizes are passed through the trochar system finally permitting a tube of 6.0–6.5mm diameter to be placed in the trachea.

Percutaneous dilatational cricothyrotomy

This is a new approach to cricothyrotomy based on the Seldinger principle which is gaining in popularity (Fig. 2.45).

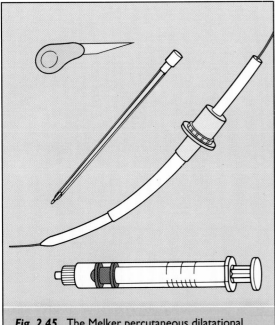

Fig. 2.45 The Melker percutaneous dilatational cricothyrotomy kit.

Technique
1 Insert an 18G cannula-over-needle into the trachea through the cricothyroid membrane and direct it caudally.
2 Confirm correct placement by aspiration of air.
3 Remove aspirating syringe and needle and pass the flexible guidewire through the cannula into the trachea. Remove the cannula leaving the guidewire in situ.
4 Make transverse incision in the skin across the guidewire entry point and extend it to pierce the cricothyroid membrane beneath.
5 Thread the dilator over the guidewire and through the membrane into the trachea.
6 Railroad a 6.0mm tube over the dilator into the trachea.
7 Secure the trachea tube in place with tape or sutures.

VENTILATION OF THE LUNGS USING BASIC LIFE SUPPORT TECHNIQUES

Effective ventilation of the lungs can be provided by Expired Air Respiration (EAR) using the mouth to mouth or mouth to nose method. This technique should be used in all apnoeic patients unless advanced equipment is immediately available.

The Mouth To Mouth Method

This method (Fig. 2.46) is preferred as a first choice by most authorities including the American Heart Association, the Resuscitation Council UK, the European, Australian, and Southern African Resuscitation Councils and the WFSA CPR Committee.

Technique
1 Place the patient in the supine position, with the head and neck aligned in the clear airway position using downward pressure on the forehead with one hand.
2 Press the thumb and forefinger of the same hand together to close the nostrils.
3 Support the chin with the other hand holding the mouth a finger breadth open.

Note: only the minimum head extension to secure a patent airway should be used in patients with suspected cervical spine injury. ■■■■■■

.....5 The rescuer, placed to the side of the patient's head, inhales, opens his own mouth wide and seals it over the victim's mouth, and blows until the chest rises as with a normal breath.

6 If inflation is difficult and the airway appears obstructed extend the head tilt further and thrust the jaw forward. Foreign body obstruction may be relieved with finger sweeps, back blows and abdominal thrusts.

7 Once inflation has occurred the rescuer removes his mouth allowing complete passive exhalation to occur in the victim, inhales again and repeats the process.

The Mouth To Nose Method

This method (Fig. 2.47) is preferred only by a minority of authorities as a first choice but it has particular advantages in certain situations, for example trismus, mandibular injury and where there are cultural objections to the mouth to mouth method.

Problems may occur with the mouth to nose method in patients with nasal obstruction and in nasal or maxillary injury.

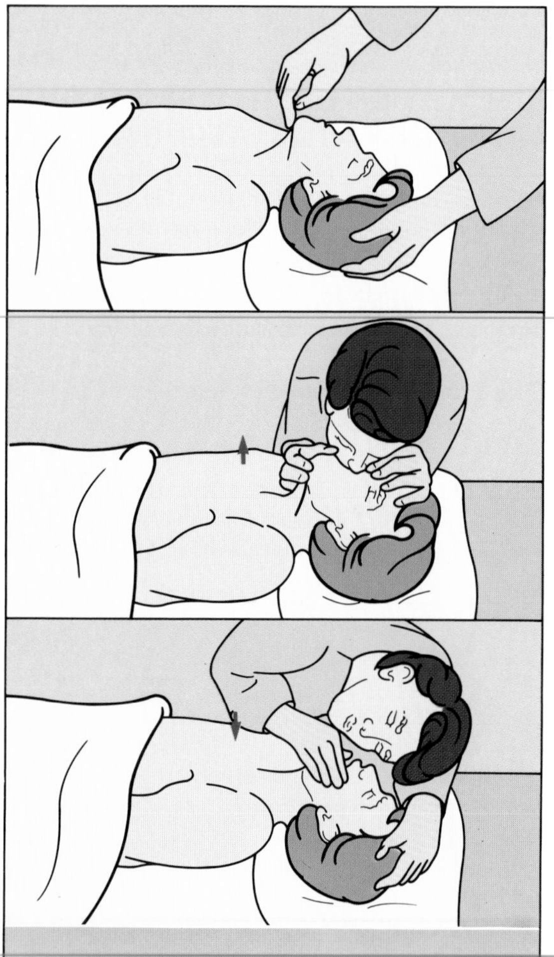

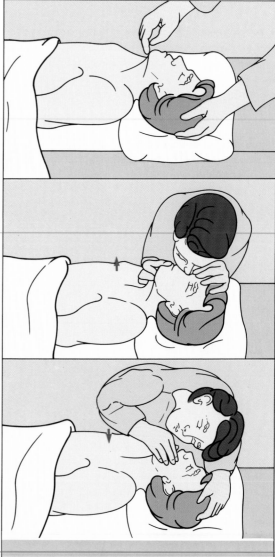

Fig. 2.46 Mouth to mouth ventilation.

Fig. 2.47 Mouth to nose ventilation.

Technique

1 The patient and rescuer are positioned as for mouth to mouth ventilation.
2 The rescuer tilts the head with a hand placed on the forehead and seals the lips with the thumb of the other hand which is placed under the chin to support it.
3 Inflation of the lungs is applied by the rescuer inhaling, sealing his mouth around the victim's nose and blowing to achieve normal inspiratory chest expansion.
4 Difficulty in inflation may occur with nasal obstruction or head/neck malalignment.
5 Passive exhalation should be ensured by opening the patient's mouth during this phase in case there is nasal obstruction.

Rate, Volumes, Flow Rates and Pressures with EAR

Rates

Respiratory rates equivalent to normal physiological rates for the patient's age should be applied during EAR. This means a rate of 10–12 breaths/min for adults, 20/min for children of 6 months to 2 years and 30/min for small infants.

Volumes

Tidal volumes slightly above normal physiological values should be the goal, ranging from 800–1000ml in adults down to 25–50ml in small infants. The chest movement expected in normal spontaneous ventilation in that particular patient is a good guide.

Flow rates

Inspiratory flow rates should mimic normal values of around 30l/min. Inflation times should be gauged to normal respiration. It is tempting to blow in too quickly. An inspiratory/expiratory ratio of 1:2 or 1:3 should be aimed at with a total time of 1.5–2.0/seconds ventilation.

Pressures

Excessive inflation pressures can occur with high flow rates, large tidal volumes and respiratory rates which do not allow sufficient time for complete exhalation. High inflation pressures (greater than 20cmH$_2$0) especially in the presence of an even slightly imperfect airway alignment lead to gastric inflation and a high probability of regurgitation and pulmonary inhalation. It has been estimated that some degree of pulmonary aspiration occurs in about 30–40 per cent of patients having EAR.

Cricoid pressure

The possibility of gastric inflation and regurgitation of stomach contents can be substantially reduced during ventilation of the unprotected airway by an assistant applying cricoid pressure (Fig. 2.48) to obstruct the lumen of the oesophagus lying posteriorly behind the larynx and in front of the cervical vertebral bodies.

Technique

1 Consistent backward pressure is applied, with the thumb and forefinger of one hand applied to either side of the cricoid cartilage.
2 Counter pressure at the back of the neck is applied with the other hand.

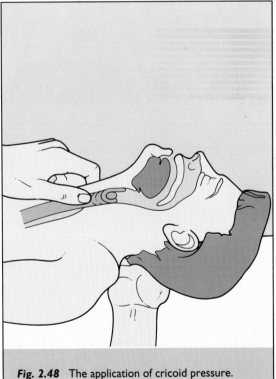

Fig. 2.48 The application of cricoid pressure.

VENTILATION OF THE LUNGS USING ADVANCED LIFE SUPPORT

Expired Air Methods Using Sample Appliances

By definition these methods are classified as advanced life support techniques as they require equipment; however, they are capable of being used by trained lay members of the public. The use of these simple inexpensive appliances, if they are readily to hand, carries a number of advantages over direct mouth to mouth or mouth to nose ventilation:

- They avoid aesthetic concern about direct contact between rescuer and victim, especially in the presence of vomit, blood, etc.
- They reduce the possibility of cross infection between rescuer and victim (see Section 1: 'Infection Hazards in Resuscitation').
- With certain appliances oxygen can be added to the expired air.
- With certain appliances airway patency is improved by an oropharyngeal tube attachment.

These appliances are of two types: the mask type and the tube/flange type.

The mask type

Expired air ventilation is applied through the port of a moulded air face-mask similar to that used in anaesthesia (Fig. 2.49). A unidirectional valve diverts the victim's expired air away from the rescuer. Certain models incorporate a nipple for attachment of an oxygen line. The mask is made of transparent material so that blood, vomit, etc., can be observed. Examples include the Laerdal Pocket Mask, the Seal Vent Easy and the MTM Resuscitator.

> **Technique**
> 1 Place the patient supine with the head and neck aligned in the clear airway position.
> 2 Apply the mask to the face using the thumb and forefingers of both hands.
> 3 Lift the angles of the jaw with the other three fingers to obtain an airtight fit in the clear airway position.
> 4 Blow into the port of the mask to inflate the patient's lungs, as in the mouth to mouth technique.
> 5 If a leak occurs at the mask–face interface, adjust the position of the thumb and forefingers slightly to obtain an airtight seal.
> 6 If an oxygen nipple is fitted and a supply is readily available, add oxygen at a flow rate of 8–10 l/min.
> 7 Alternatively a tube from an oxygen source can be placed in the rescuer's mouth to enhance the inspired oxygen concentration.

The tube flange type

Expired air ventilation is applied to a tube with a flange to seal the lips and a short oropharyngeal airway (Fig. 2.50). Certain models include a unidirectional valve to divert the victim's expired air away from the rescuer, and some have a nose clip included as part of the equipment. Examples include the Hi Tilt Airway, the Brook Airway and the Safar "S" Airway.

> **Technique**
> 1 Place the patient supine with the head and neck aligned in the clear airway position.
> 2 Introduce the distal end of the tube into the patient's mouth, being careful not to displace the tongue backwards.
> 3 Lifting the angles of the jaw on both sides ....

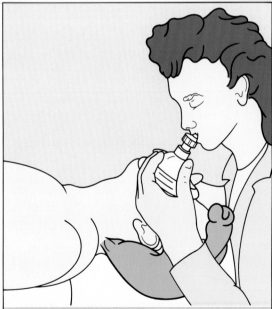

Fig. 2.49 Ventilation using the mouth to mask technique (Laerdal pocket mask with oxygen nipple and unidirectional valve).

.... with the little and ring fingers, seal the flange over the patient's lips with the thumbs and forefingers, and compress the nostrils between the base of both thumbs (use the nose clip if provided).

4 Blow into the proximal end of the tube to inflate the patient's lungs, as in the mouth to mouth technique.

The Self-Inflating Bag/valve Device

The self-inflating bag/valve device is designed to inflate the patient's lungs with room air or an air–oxygen mixture if an oxygen supply is readily available. It has a clear advantage over expired air techniques in that a higher inspired oxygen-concentration can be provided. However, use of the self-inflating bag/valve does require much more training and expertise which is not as easily acquired as is often supposed.

The self-inflating bag is fitted at one end with an inlet valve to entrain air or an air–oxygen mixture

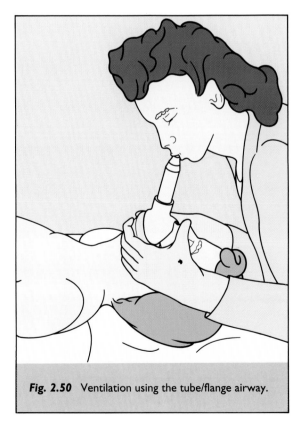

Fig. 2.50 Ventilation using the tube/flange airway.

into the bag as it reflates during the expiratory phase. During compression of the bag the air or air–oxygen mixture inflates the patient's lungs through the patient valve. This valve diverts the expired air into the atmosphere. The valve may be attached to a face-mask, endotracheal tube, tracheostomy tube, laryngeal mask, PLTA or Combitube via a 15mm fitting.

Addition of oxygen

Oxygen can be added to the bag either via a nipple, a reservoir bag or a length of reservoir tubing. Best results are achieved using a reservoir bag (less bulky) or a length of reservoir tubing (Fig. 2.51). With these additions inspired oxygen concentrations of 90 per cent can be achieved with oxygen flow rates of 8–10 l/min. The inlet valve of bags incorporating an oxygen reservoir bag or tubing must be so designed that air will be entrained if the oxygen supply runs out. The addition of oxygen through a nipple on the bag, without a reservoir, is much less efficient. To achieve a high inspired oxygen concentration the flow rates of oxygen must be comparable with the inspiratory flow rate (circa 25–30 l/min). Such high flow rates over-fill the bag during inspiration, jamming the patient valve in the inspiratory position and preventing expiration through the valve. If no reservoir system is available, the added oxygen flow rate must not exceed 5–6 l/min (which will only achieve inspired oxygen concentrations of 40–50 per cent).

Positive end expiratory pressure

Positive end expiratory pressure (PEEP) can be provided with a self-inflating bag if a special PEEP valve

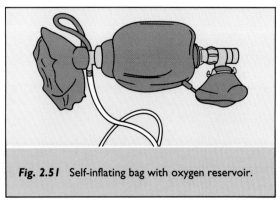

Fig. 2.51 Self-inflating bag with oxygen reservoir.

is attached at the patient end (Fig. 2.52). PEEP can be applied most effectively if the bag is attached to an endotracheal tube rather than a face-mask. PEEP is particularly valuable in patients with pulmonary oedema due to heart failure, burns, aspiration or inhalation of irritant chemicals, and in victims of near drowning.

Technique

1 Place the patient supine with the head, neck and jaw in the clear airway position.
2 Apply the mask to the patient's face to achieve an airtight fit.
3 Hold the face-mask firmly in place with the thumb and forefinger forming a collar around the circumference of the mask near the port for attachment to the patient valve.
4 Use the third, ring and little finger to support the jaw and thrust it forwards to maintain a clear airway.
5 An airtight seal is achieved by pressing the thumb and forefinger towards the other three fingers holding the jaw. (Fig. 2.53).
6 Compressing the bag inflates the patient's lungs.

Care should be taken not to generate excessively high flow rates as this will result in high pharyngeal pressures and gastric inflation, regurgitation and pulmonary aspiration. Cricoid pressure by an assistant reduces the chances of this complication.

7 Release of the bag results in refilling and simultaneous passive exhalation through the expiratory port of the patient valve.
8 Add oxygen (8–10l/min if a reservoir is fitted; 5l/min if a nipple only is fitted) if available.
9 As soon as tracheal intubation or laryngeal mask insertion has been accomplished the bag is fitted to the tube and ventilation can be handed over to a less skilled assistant who is instructed to compress and release with an inspiratory/expiratory ratio of 1:2 or 1:3, achieving normal chest movements at a normal rate for the victim's age.

Selection of a self-inflating bag

The points to look for in the selection of a self-inflating bag unit include:

- Material of the bag: this should have a satisfactory "feel", should not be able to absorb anaesthetic vapours or noxious gases, and should remain effective in use over a wide variation in temperature. Foam-filled units should not be capable of undetectable disintegration inside, with the inherent danger of inflating fragments of foam into the patient's lungs. During reflation the bag should have sufficient recoil to activate a drawover anaesthetic system.
- Valve function: both inlet and patient valves should be of robust construction, competent, and simple in operation and incapable of sticking in one position. They should be easy to take apart, clean and reassemble. Incorrect reassembly should be impossible.

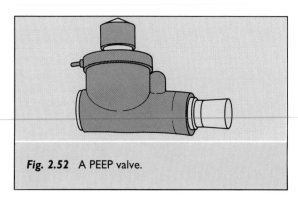

Fig. 2.52 A PEEP valve.

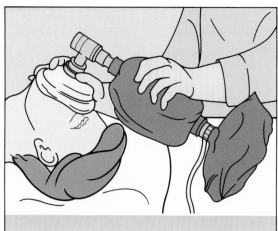

Fig. 2.53 Use of a self-inflating bag and mask.

- The inlet valve should be capable of being fitted with a filter (to exclude noxious gases) and an oxygen reservoir bag.
- The patient valve should have standard ISO (International Standards Organisation) fittings (15mm) for attachment to a face-mask or endotracheal tube.
- The bag should be supplied in a convenient carrying case capable of including other relevant items such as oro- and nasopharyngeal airways and equipment for endotracheal intubation.

Effective models include those made by Vitalograph, Laerdal, Ambu, etc.

Manually Triggered Oxygen-powered Resuscitators

These devices are powered by a high pressure (414pKa/60psi) oxygen source connected to a valve which is manually operated to open to provide lung inflation via a face-mask, endotracheal tube or cricothyrotomy tube (Fig. 2.54).

The advantage of this system over the self-inflating bag is that both hands may be used by the operator to apply the mask to the face and control the head, neck and jaw in the clear airway position. Many units also have a demand trigger mode for oxygen therapy for patients who revert to spontaneous respiration after resuscitation. The disadvantage of the system is that the lack of "feel" during the inspiratory phase makes it easy to cause gastric inflation if airway control is not perfect. To meet the

recommendations of the American Heart Association and other bodies, inspiratory flow rates should not exceed 40l/min and the valve should incorporate a blow-off device at 60cmH$_2$O (30cmH$_2$O in children). Manually triggered oxygen-powered resuscitators should only be used by trained paramedical personnel and not by relatively unskilled members of the lay public or first-aiders.

> **Technique**
> 1. Using both thumbs and forefingers apply the face-mask with attached valve to the face.
> 2. Support the jaw using the other three fingers of both hands, as with mouth to mask ventilation.
> 3. Inflation is achieved by depressing the valve trigger with a thumb and watching the chest rise.
> 4. Releasing the trigger at the end of inflation is followed by passive expiration.

Automatic Resuscitators

Automatic resuscitators are small, portable ventilators designed for use in the field and while the patient is in transport. They are powered by compressed oxygen at 310-414 pKa (45-60psi) and cycled either by a fluid logic arrangement or by electronic circuitry using a small battery. Their versatility and complexity varies from model to model. More complex models are termed transport ventilators. Ventilation may be applied through a face-mask, laryngeal mask or endotracheal tube or other airway adjunct. When a face-mask is used, two hands are available for application of the mask to the face and for airway alignment, which represents an advantage over the self-inflating bag. However, as with the manually triggered oxygen-powered resuscitator, "feel" associated with lung inflation is lost and meticulous care must be taken to ensure airway patency throughout, otherwise gastric inflation will occur. Automatic resuscitators perform best when attached to an endotracheal tube.

Cycling mechanism

The cycling mechanism should be volume-preset and time-cycled. Pressure-cycled devices are of no value during chest compressions as they cycle with each compression.

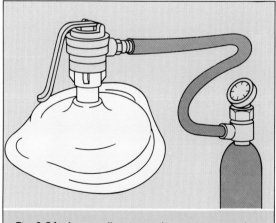

Fig. 2.54 A manually triggered oxygen powered resuscitator.

Some models incorporate the option of an air-oxygen mix device which allows air to be entrained in certain suitable cases and conserves the oxygen supply.

> ### Technique
> 1 Place the patient in the supine position with the head, neck and jaw aligned in the clear airway position.
> 2 Adjust the control knobs to a suitable tidal volume, inspiration/expiration (I/E) ratio and air-oxygen mix, and select the blow-off valve setting and PEEP valve as appropriate.
> 3 Turn on the oxygen supply.
> 4 Apply the mask with the attached patient valve to the face using both hands to achieve an airtight fit with jaw support. Alternatively attach the patient valve to the laryngeal mask or endotracheal tube connector.
> 5 Inspiration and expiration occur rhythmically and automatically.
> 6 Continue to ensure airway patency breath-by-breath throughout when a face-mask is used.

Selection of an Automatic Resuscitator

The points to look for in selection include:

The technical specification of the control module
Dimensions, weight and strength.
Driving gas pressure and consumption.
Availability of air–oxygen mixture facility.
Filter protection facility on air–oxygen mix models.
Range of respiratory rate and minute volume.
Inspiratory flow rate should not exceed 40l/min.
Cycling mechanism should be volume-preset and time-cycled.
Variable inspiratory/expiratory ratio facility.

The technical specification of the patient valve
Standard ISO connections for mask, endotracheal tube and scavenging devices.
Robust manufacture, competent, simple in operation and incapable of sticking in one position.
Easily dismantled, cleaned and reassembled without the possibility of error.
PEEP valve facility.
Possibility of spontaneous ventilation without significant resistance if the resuscitator fails.

General points
Ease of use and simplicity of controls.
Ability to withstand rough treatment in clinical practice.
Ability to be used with CPR.
Carrying case with room for related equipment for airway maintenance, for example oro- and nasopharyngeal airways and endotracheal intubation set.

Suitable models
The Pneupac Rescupac and Parapac (fluid logic control; Figs 2.55 & 2.56).
The Drager Oxylog Resuscitator (fluid logic control).
The Unimed Resuscitator (fluid logical control).
The Uni-Vent Resuscitator (electronic control; Fig. 2.57).

Transcricoid jet ventilator
This is an invasive method which may be suitable in patients in whom endotracheal intubation is not possible.

Oxygen (or an air–oxygen mixture) at 310–414pKa (45–60psi) is insufflated through high pressure tubing connected to a 14G cannula introduced into the trachea through the cricothyroid membrane. The inspiratory phase is achieved by controlled release of the oxygen supply using a manually operated trigger valve until the chest rises.

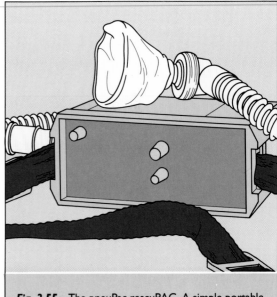

Fig. 2.55 The pneuPac rescuPAC. A simple portable automatic resuscitator with minimal operator variables.

Technique

I Place the patient supine with the head and neck extended. Check that there is no upper airway obstruction.

2 Make a small skin incision (3mm) over the cricothyroid membrane. Introduce two 14G cannulae over needle into the trachea through the cricothyroid membrane.

3 Connect the high pressure tubing from the trigger valve and the oxygen source to one of the cannulae using a Luerlok system.

4 Inflation of the lungs is produced by manual compression of the trigger which is immediately released as the chest rises.

5 Passive expiration follows.

Expiration occurs passively through the larynx, mouth and nose, and the system must not be used in patients with upper airway obstruction which would prevent expiration.

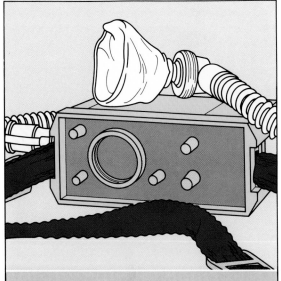

Fig. 2.56 The pneuPac paraPAC. A portable automatic resuscitator with independently variable frequency and tidal volume and inflation pressure monitor.

SUPPORT OF THE CIRCULATION

The circulation may be temporarily supported after cardiac arrest by Basic or Advanced Life Support measures.

Recognition of Cardiac Arrest

Three signs only are necessary to confirm cardiac arrest: unconsciousness, absence of a palpable pulse in a large artery and a death-like appearance.

Unconsciousness

The patient loses consciousness about 15–20 seconds after sudden cardiac arrest.

Absence of a palpable arterial pulse in a large artery

The carotid or femoral arteries are the most suitable vessels to palpate. The common carotid artery lies between the larynx and the sternocleidomastoid strap muscle running between the manubrium sternum and clavicle to the mastoid process behind the ear (Fig. 2.58).

More peripheral pulses are misleading as they may be difficult to feel in hypovolaemia even when there is still a spontaneous, small cardiac output.

In infants the brachial artery is preferred as the carotid may be more difficult to feel and palpation attempts may interfere with airway patency.

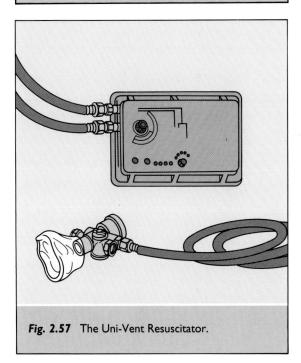

Fig. 2.57 The Uni-Vent Resuscitator.

A death-like appearance

The patient's colour will be either very blue (asphyxia), very grey (primary cardiac arrest) or very pale (hypovolaemia and hypothermia).

Other signs may accompany cardiac arrest such as apnoea or agonal gasping respirations and dilated pupils (Fig. 2.59). However time should not be wasted confirming these signs before beginning resuscitation. Dilated pupils do not occur in every case and may be precluded by drugs, previous eye surgery, etc.

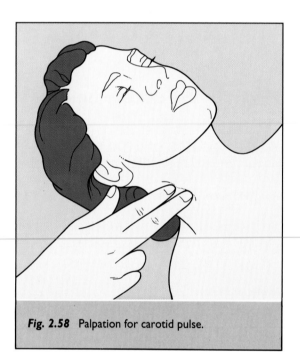

Fig. 2.58 Palpation for carotid pulse.

External Chest Compressions

External chest compressions (ECC) are a basic life support measure which can be successfully taught to and applied by members of the lay public as well as health care professionals; they consist of rhythmical compressions applied over the lower half of the sternum. The term "external chest compressions" is much preferred to the term "external cardiac massage" as it is a more accurate description of the procedure.

Mechanism of Action

There is still considerable academic debate as to the best method of application of chest compressions in combination with artificial ventilation. There is much evidence to support the value of creating an intermittent raised intrathoracic pressure during chest compressions (thoracic pump effect), but these considerations do not apply during basic life support using the unintubated airway. Under such conditions ECC is thought to produce a circulation by virtue of intermittent compression of the heart between the spinal column and back of the sternum, and it is assumed that there is at least some continuing function of the valves of the heart (cardiac pump effect; Fig. 2.60). Although some doubt has been cast on the latter statement by experimental work, the countless cases of recorded clinical success with simple ECC and mouth to mouth ventilation do support this hypothesis.

In any case ECCs provide at best a very modest cardiac output (20–40 per cent of normal values) and it is vital that they should be continued without

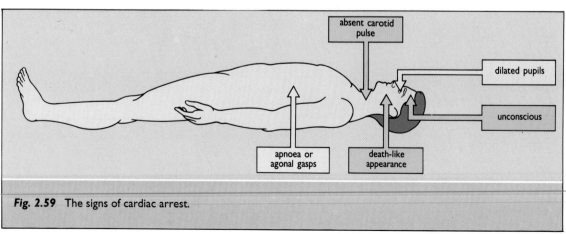

Fig. 2.59 The signs of cardiac arrest.

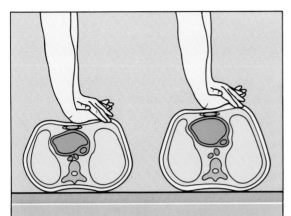

Fig. 2.60 Compression of the heart between the spinal column and back of the sternum.

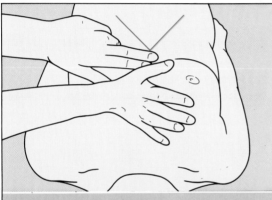

Fig. 2.61 Location of the compression point using two fingers placed above the xiphisternum.

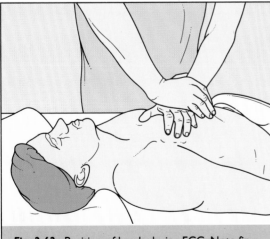

Fig. 2.62 Position of hands during ECC. Note fingers off ribs.

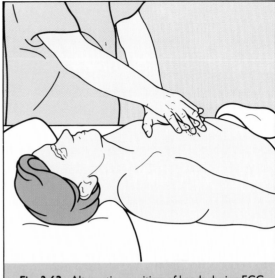

Fig. 2.63 Alternative position of hands during ECC (fingers intertwined). Note fingers off ribs.

interruption for more than a very few seconds (e.g. endotracheal intubation, i.v. cannulation), otherwise it is difficult to re-establish a circulation and irreversible cerebral and other organ damage will occur.

Technique

1 Place the patient supine on a firm surface.
2 Elevate the legs, if possible, to improve venous return.
3 Kneeling by the side of the patient's chest locate the site for compression using one of the following methods:
   • Place two fingers on the xiphisternum and place the heel of the other hand above them on the sternum in the midline (Fig. 2.61).
   • Place the centre of the heel of the hand in the midline on a point at the junction of the upper two-thirds and lower third of the distance between the manubrium and xiphisternum.
   • Place the centre of the heel of the hand on the sternum at the nipple line.
4 Place the other hand on top of the hand located correctly on the sternum either intertwining the fingers or grasping the wrist with the thumb. The fingers should be kept off the ribs to avoid rib fractures (Figs 2.62 & 2.63). ▪▪▪▪▪

5 With the elbows straight and shoulders placed over the patient's chest, apply rhythmical compressions using a stroke of 4–5cm (Fig. 2.64).

6 The compression rate should be at least 80–100/min and the compression phase should occupy 50 per cent of the cycle.

The praecordial thump

The praecordial thump has been advocated as a method of cardioverting a recently arrested heart, and there are several documented reports of success in converting ventricular fibrillation and asystole to sinus rhythm. There have also been some reports of reversion of ventricular fibrillation to asystole following the thump.

The manoeuvre should be reserved for cases where the arrest is literally witnessed by the rescuer and should be followed by ECC and EAR if not immediately successful.

Technique

I Place the patient in a supine position.

2 With the ulnar aspect of the clenched fist deliver a blow to the sternum at the junction of the upper two-thirds and the lower third of the distance between the manubrium and xiphisternum in the midline (Fig. 2.65).

Fist pacing

Cases have been reported of patients with witnessed asystole who have responded to a series of praecordial thumps which have had the effect of acting as a mechanical pacemaker. If a single praecordial thump is temporarily effective but the patient reverts to clinical arrest it is worth trying a series of thumps at a rate of 60–80/min to see if the patient responds by improvement in colour, return of spontaneous breathing, improvement in level of consciousness, etc. If there is no sign of improvement in 30 seconds then formal CPR should be instituted immediately.

Cough CPR

It has been demonstrated in certain patients that spontaneous rhythmical coughing started at the moment of arrest can generate sufficient cardiac output to maintain consciousness for 1–2 minutes. This

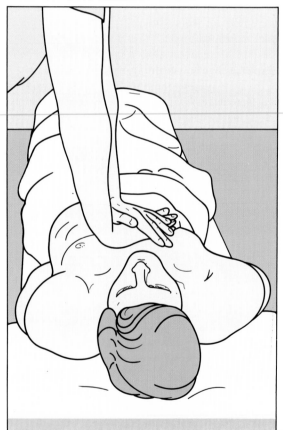

Fig. 2.64 Application of external chest compressions.

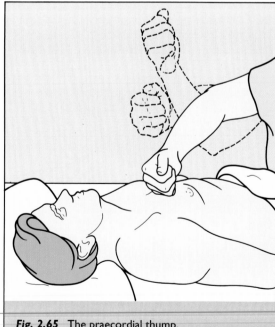

Fig. 2.65 The praecordial thump.

clearly demonstrates the thoracic pump effect of intermittent high intrathoracic pressures. The technique has little practical application — the patient must either be trained to watch his own ECG monitor with rapt attention or the attendant must order him to cough immediately an arrest occurs and before consciousness is lost 15 seconds later. At best the technique buys 1–2 minutes of time.

Selected patients at risk might be taught to cough hard, with deep breaths in between, at the rate of once per second if they feel that their heart has stopped but, if there is no cardiac arrest, potential harm could be done by inducing hypoxia, brachycardia, syncope or even ventricular fibrillation.

Active compression decompression (ACD)

Following successful outcome after resuscitation using chest compressions with a domestic drain plunger, early experimental work in animals and humans has confirmed that active compression and decompression of the chest wall may well promise to produce better cardiac output, systolic blood pressure and end tidal CO_2 values during resuscitation when compared to standard ECC.

Ambu have developed a device (the Ambu Cardio pump) based on the suction drain plunger principle which is currently undergoing clinical trials in several centres worldwide.

The device consists of a vacuum cup some 15cm in diameter which is applied to the patient's chest in the same position as the hands in standard ECC (Fig. 2.66) The same compression technique and rate is used as for standard ECC. Active Decompression is achieved by pulling up on the device between compressions. The vacuum cup sticks to the chest and transfers a lifting force to the lower part of the rib cage. A gauge indicating both compression and decompression forces is incorporated into the handle of the device.

Technique
I Apply the Cardiopump to the patient's sternum with the centre of the pump at the junction of the upper two thirds and lower one third of the sternum (Fig. 2.67). ▪▪▪▪▪▪

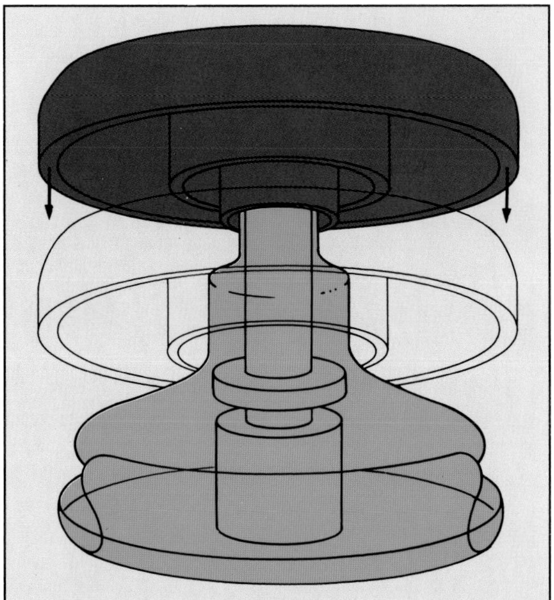

Fig. 2.66 The Ambu Cardio pump

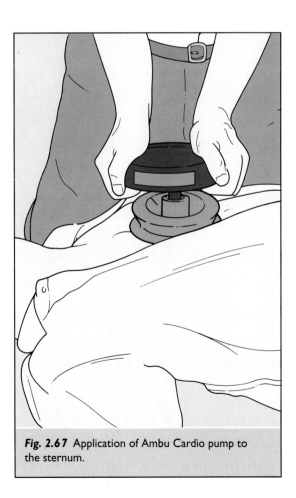

Fig. 2.67 Application of Ambu Cardio pump to the sternum.

......2 Apply rhythmical compressions at a rate of 80–100/min with a stroke of 4–5cm using a force of 27–41kg (60–90lb) (in adults) (Fig. 2.68.a).

3 Between compressions pull up on the cardiopump handle achieve active decompression by elevating the lower rib cage using a force of 9kg (20lb) (in adults) (see Fig. 2.68.b).

4 Ventilations are interposed using the same sequence as with standard CPR.

Open Chest Cardiac Massage

The heart can be massaged through the open chest to produce an output which is often superior to that generated by external chest compressions. However, this advanced life support technique can only be applied by physicians trained in the appropriate surgical skills, with suitable facilities, and there is an inevitable delay in restoring a cardiac output while the chest is opened. There are therefore only certain specific indications for using the open chest method in preference to external chest compressions.

Indications for open chest cardiac massage
- Cardiac arrest during cardiothoracic surgery.
- Cardiac arrest due to cardiac tamponade.
- Cardiac arrest due to major intrathoracic or intra-abdominal haemorrhage.
- Cardiac arrest due to pulmonary embolism when open pulmonary embolectomy is planned.
- Cardiac arrest due to hypothermia when direct rewarming of the heart with saline is planned.

Technique
1 The patient should be intubated and ventilated with intermittent positive pressure.
2 An incision is made through skin and the intercostal muscles in the fifth intercostal space from near the midline to the midaxillary line (Fig. 2.69).
3 A nick is made in the pleura with a scalpel and the incision continued with scissors or blunt dissection, carefully avoiding the lung and heart beneath.
4 A self-retaining rib spreader is inserted.
5 The operator's left hand compresses the heart between the fingers posteriorly on the left ventricle and the thumb anteriorly on the right ventricle (Fig. 2.70). Rhythmical compressions are continued at the rate of 60/min or as dictated by cardiac filling. ....

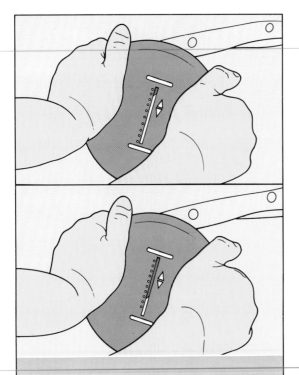

Fig. 2.68 Compression (above)and decompression (below) with Ambu Cardio pump.

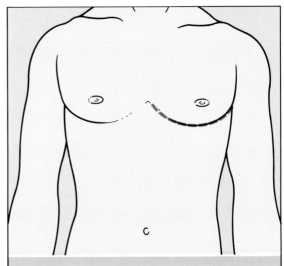

Fig. 2.69 Incision in left fifth intercostal space for open chest cardiac massage.

......6 The pericardium is opened in cases of cardiac tamponade and for intracardiac drug injection and direct application of defibrillator paddles.

7 Bleeding vessels in the thorax are controlled or clamped as indicated.

8 Abdominal bleeding may be temporarily controlled by compression of the descending aorta while abdominal laparotomy is performed for definitive haemorrhage control.

Extracorporeal Circulation

Cardiopulmonary bypass using an extracorporeal circulation may be used in certain patients with cardiorespiratory arrest who have conditions amenable to immediate cardiac surgery, such as pulmonary embolectomy, coronary artery bypass grafting and valve replacement. Details of this specialized technique are outside the scope of this handbook.

Intra-aortic Balloon Counter Pulsation

This technique may be used to support patients with failing hearts in imminent danger of arrest after cardiac surgery, or where the cause may be amenable to cardiac surgery. The technique is quicker to estab-

lish than full cardiopulmonary bypass but likewise requires highly specialized equipment and expert personnel.

A special balloon is introduced into the aorta and inflation is linked to the heartbeat by electronic control from the electrocardiograph. The balloon inflates during diastole and deflates during systole, so increasing the diastolic pressure (and thus coronary artery flow) without detracting from the systolic pressure.

Again, details of this specialized technique are outside the scope of this handbook.

COORDINATION OF VENTILATION AND CHEST COMPRESSIONS

One rescuer method (BLS)

With one rescuer two ventilations, each occupying 1.5-2.0 seconds, should be followed by 15 compressions at the rate of 80-100/min (Fig. 2.71). This sequence is designed to minimize time wasted by the rescuer re-positioning between the chest and the face.

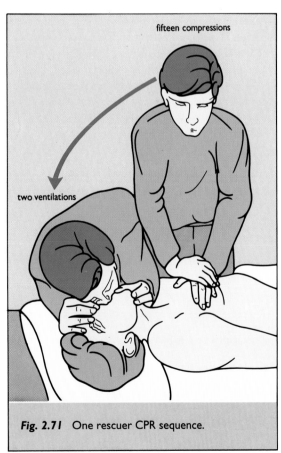

Fig. 2.71 One rescuer CPR sequence.

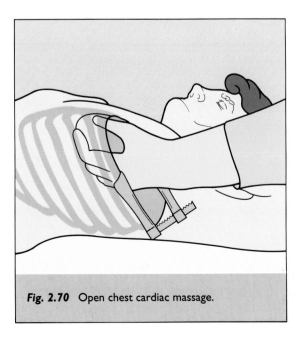

Fig. 2.70 Open chest cardiac massage.

47

Two rescuer method (BLS)

With two trained rescuers a sequence of one ventilation to five compressions should be followed. The first rescuer should give one ventilation over 1.5–2.0 seconds, followed by the second rescuer giving five compressions at a rate of 80–100/min and then pausing for 1.5–2.0 seconds for a further ventilation, and so on (Fig. 2.72). This sequence is near the physiological norm. It is helpful if the rescuer doing chest compressions calls out the rhythm.

Performing external chest compressions is hard work and if the rescuer in that role tires he should change places with the rescuer providing ventilation. The best way to do this minimizing interruption of chest compressions is, at the end of a breath, for the ventilator to move in front of the compressor and take over chest compressions. Simultaneously the compressor moves back and goes behind his colleague in time to provide a breath after five compressions have been completed (Fig. 2.73).

Two rescuers with an intubated patient

When the patient is intubated the sequence may be modified slightly to take some advantage of the suspected benefits of intermittent high intrathoracic pressures during chest compressions which enhance cardiac filling and output (the thoracic pump effect). In this case, chest compressions should continue at 80–100/min with a ventilation superimposed at every five compressions. Because the patient's airway is secured by the cuffed tracheal tube there is no danger of pulmonary aspiration. There is however a potential danger of alveolar rupture due to barotrauma.

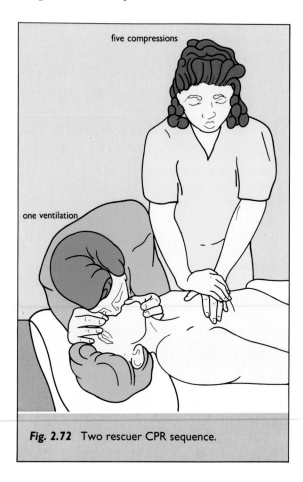

Fig. 2.72 Two rescuer CPR sequence.

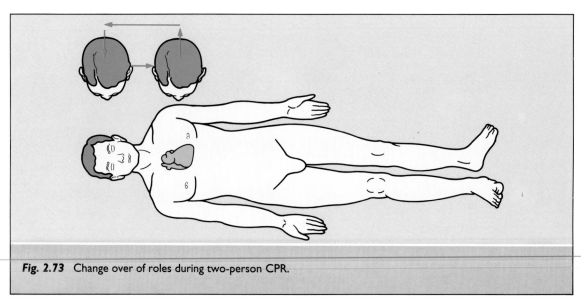

Fig. 2.73 Change over of roles during two-person CPR.

RESTORATION OF THE SPONTANEOUS HEARTBEAT

For definitive restoration of the spontaneous heart-beat ideally it is necessary to obtain the electrocardiogram (ECG) of the arrested heart. Once this has been established then precise treatment can be insti-gated using electrical defibrillation or drug therapy, or a combination of both. Since treatment is to be based almost entirely on the ECG diagnosis, it is essential that this trace be recorded without artefact.

RECORDING AN ECG TRACE

In a cardiac arrest or potential cardiac arrest, the ECG trace should be obtained using either ECG defibrillator paddle electrodes or adhesive chest electrodes.

Electrode Placement

ECG defibrillator paddle electrodes

ECG defibrillator paddle or large adhesive electrodes should be placed in the Lead II position over the apex of the heart (+ve) and at the right sternal border just beneath the right clavicle (-ve) (Figs 2.74 and 2.75). Firm steady pressure should be applied when using paddle electrodes to ensure good contact without artefact. Misleading artefacts resembling ventricular fibrillation may occur with shaking hands or vibrating conditions, for example during ambulance or helicopter travel. It is good practice to use conductive pads or electrode jelly to improve the quality of the trace, but this is not essential under ideal conditions. Large adhesive electrodes eliminate artefacts.

The ECG defibrillator paddle electrodes (see Fig. 2.75) are marked "apex" and "sternum" to indicate their correct position. If the paddles are inadvertently reversed then the trace will be "upside down", which will be of no consequence in ventricular fibrillation or asystole and should be recognized easily in normal sinus rhythm.

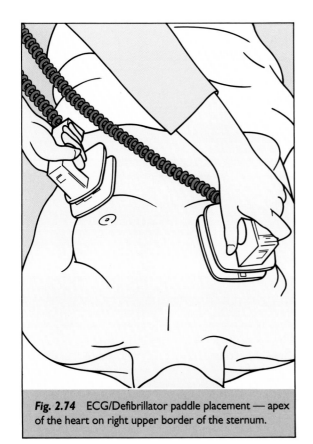

Fig. 2.74 ECG/Defibrillator paddle placement — apex of the heart on right upper border of the sternum.

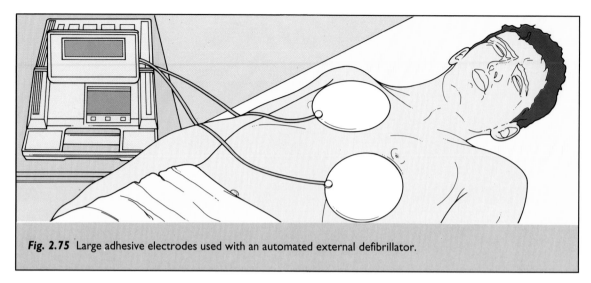

Fig. 2.75 Large adhesive electrodes used with an automated external defibrillator.

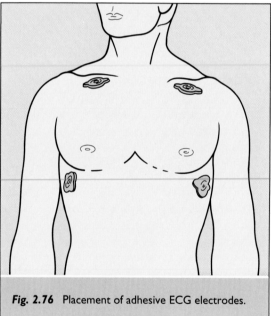

Fig. 2.76 Placement of adhesive ECG electrodes.

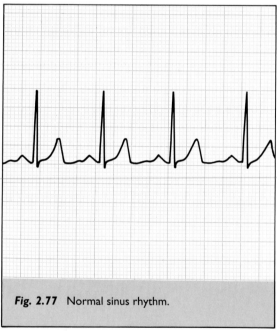

Fig. 2.77 Normal sinus rhythm.

Adhesive chest electrodes

Standard adhesive chest electrodes should be placed in the conventional three lead positions below the left clavicle, below the right clavicle and over the apex of the heart (Fig. 2.76).

- Lead I records the ECG between the electrodes placed below the left (+ve) and the right (-ve) clavicle.
- Lead II records the ECG between the electrodes placed over the apex of the heart (+ve) and the right clavicle (-ve).
- Lead III records the ECG between the electrodes placed over the apex of the heart (+ve) and the left clavicle (-ve).

If a fourth lead (earth or ground) is provided it can be located almost anywhere but is generally placed just outside and below the right nipple (equivalent position to the apex of the heart on the right side).

Adhesive chest electrodes should be of the pre-gelled type. To reduce confusion in the emergency situation they are attached to colour-coded leads by "popper" studs or "clothes pegs" chips.

THE NORMAL ECG

ECG in normal sinus rhythm is shown in Figure 2.77.
• P wave is due to atrial depolarization.
• QRS complex is due to ventricular depolarization.
• T wave is due to ventricular repolarization.
The PR interval should not exceed 0.2 seconds, and the QRS complex should not exceed 0.12 seconds.

Interpretation of the ECG

The ECG should be analyzed for:
• Rate.
• Rhythm.
• Site of dominant pacemaker.
• Configuration of the P wave.
• The PR interval.
• Configuration of the QRS complex.

ECG RHYTHMS ASSOCIATED WITH CARDIAC ARREST

Three ECG patterns are associated with cardiac arrest:
• Ventricular fibrillation.
• Ventricular asystole.
• Electromechanical dissociation.

Ventricular Fibrillation

Ventricular fibrillation (VF) is the most common mechanism causing cardiac arrest in primary myocardial ischaemia. For a cardiac output to occur, the tiny ventricular muscle fibres must contract and relax together in a coordinated manner. In VF this coordination is completely lost and the fibres contract individually in a random fashion. Thus one fibre may be contracting while its neighbour is relaxing. As a result, the ventricles as a whole do not eject blood and the cardiac output is zero.

Ventricular fibrillation produces a completely disorganized ECG trace, without any rhythm or pattern resembling any form of coordinated contraction. To the naked eye the heart appears to be quivering and has been described as feeling "like a bag of worms".

At the onset of VF the muscle fibres are usually still contracting and this is briskly demonstrated by high amplitude deflections on the ECG. This is known as coarse ventricular fibrillation (Fig. 2.78).

If the VF is left untreated the muscle fibre contraction rapidly deteriorates and the deflections on ECG are reduced in amplitude. This is known as fine ventricular fibrillation (Fig. 2.79). VF is defined as deflections with an amplitude greater than 1mm (calibration 1cm/mV).

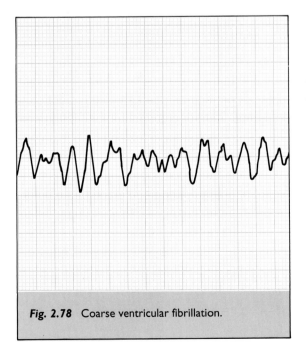

Fig. 2.78 Coarse ventricular fibrillation.

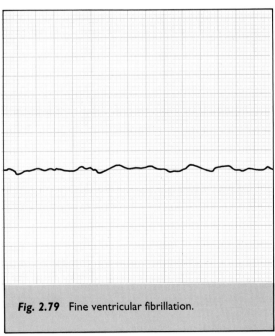

Fig. 2.79 Fine ventricular fibrillation.

Coarse VF is likely to respond to speedy electrical defibrillation. Fine VF is much less likely to respond to defibrillation. It can, on occasions, be converted back to coarse VF by the stimulant effect of adrenaline (epinephrine), and subsequent defibrillation attempts may be successful.

Left untreated, ventricular fibrillation ultimately fades to asystole as the individual fibres cease contracting altogether.

The ECG pattern of VF may be confused with artefacts resulting from electrical AC interference or from movement of the electrodes or leads, resulting in poor connections. Before finally interpreting the trace, ensure that the apparatus is electrically sound with satisfactory earthing (grounding) arrangements, that the lead connections are secure and that there is good electrical contact at the patient/electrode interface. Fine ventricular fibrillation may appear to be asystole in one of the ECG leads. Check the appearance in other leads and if in doubt treat as VF. The urgency of early defibrilation cannot be overemphasised and initial defibrilation attempts should take precedencce over other resuscitation efforts. Treatment of ventricular fibrillation is described on p.66.

Ventricular Asystole

In asystole there is no contraction of any of the ventricular muscle fibres. The rhythm is sometimes termed "cardiac death" and may occur as a primary event, or follow unsuccessfully treated VF or electromechanical dissociation.

The ECG shows a complete absence of ventricular electrical activity. On occasion P waves may occur (Fig. 2.80).

Asystole is associated with a miserable prognosis on most occasions. Treatment is described on p.68.

The ECG of asystole is often described as "a straight line". If the trace appears to be an absolutely straight line, check that the proper connections between the apparatus, the leads and the electrodes have been made and that the gain has been turned up. Asystole is not represented by an absolutely straight line in the early phases after onset, and such a trace should be viewed with suspicion before arriving at a final diagnosis.

Electromechanical Dissociation

Electromechanical dissociation (EMD) is a condition in which the patient is pulseless, with no cardiac output, but ventricular electrical activity continues. The ventricular electrical activity may initially resemble a relatively normal QRS complex, but this soon becomes very spread out and bizarre looking (Fig. 2.81).

EMD usually carries a poor prognosis and deteriorates to asystole. On occasion, however, the arrhythmia may be associated with a correctable problem such as cardiac tamponade, tension pneumothorax, hypoxia, acidosis or hypovolaemia. A less correctable cause is pulmonary embolism.

The treatment should be directed at searching for and relieving the cause and restoring spontaneous activity with adrenaline and other cardiac stimulants; it is described on p.69.

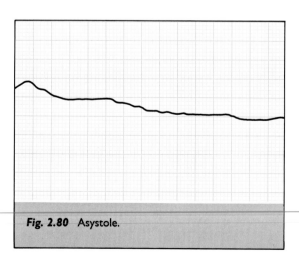

Fig. 2.80 Asystole.

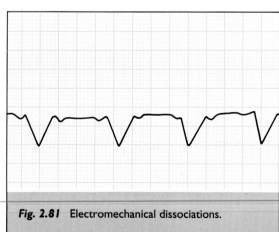

Fig. 2.81 Electromechanical dissociations.

LIFE-THREATENING ECG RHYTHMS

Certain ECG rhythms should be regarded as potentially leading to imminent cardiac arrest, and they require urgent treatment and correction.

Ventricular Tachycardia

Ventricular tachycardia (VT) is defined as occurring when three or more contractions of ventricular origin arise in succession at a rate greater than 100/min (Fig. 2.82). The rate usually lies between 150 and 220/min, and the rhythm is usually regular but may, on occasion, be irregular in parts.

P waves are not usually visible except at slower rates and they then are rarely related to the ventricular activity (atrioventricular dissociation). Occasionally a fixed P/QRS relationship does exist when retrograde ventricle to atrium conduction occurs. The QRS section is spread and occupies more than 0.12 seconds. Frequently the shape of the trace is bizarre with notching.

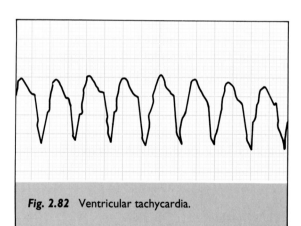

Fig. 2.82 Ventricular tachycardia.

Ventricular tachycardia is a life-threatening rhythm. The adequacy of the cardiac output depends principally on two factors:
- The degree of myocardial dysfunction giving rise to the arrhythmia.
- The rate which determines cardiac filling during diastole.

These factors determine whether the cardiac output is adequate to maintain sufficient perfusion of the vital organs. Immediate treatment varies according to whether perfusion of the brain is sufficient to maintain consciousness.

Bradycardia

Bradycardia is defined as a heart rate of less than 60/min. It may arise in conjunction with a number of ECG patterns:
- Sinus bradycardia.
- First degree atrioventricular (AV) block.
- Second degree AV block — Types I and II.
- Third degree AV block.

The treatment of the bradycardias is described on pp.70-72.

Sinus bradycardia
Sinus bradycardia is characterized by an ECG pattern of normal regular rhythm and morphology, but with an unusually long gap between the T wave and the origin of the succeeding P wave (Fig. 2.83).

First degree AV block
First degree AV block shows a regular slow rhythm with a normal QRS shape and duration but with a PR interval extended beyond 0.2 seconds (Fig. 2.84).

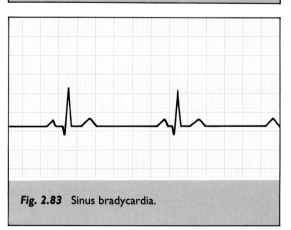

Fig. 2.83 Sinus bradycardia.

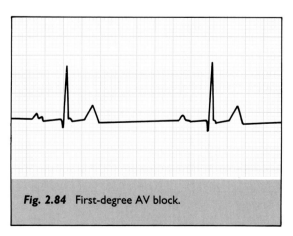

Fig. 2.84 First-degree AV block.

Second degree AV block – Type I

This type of block is also known as the Wenckebach phenomenon. The dysrhythmia is characterized by a slow regular atrial rate with an increasing PR interval until finally a P wave is not followed by a QRS complex. The process is then repeated over a series of P waves followed by QRS complexes, but with an increasing PR interval which extends, beat by beat, until once again a QRS complex is missed. Thus apparent "bursts" of QRS complexes occur (usually three to five) which are followed by a ventricular pause (Fig. 2.85).

Second degree AV block – Type II

The type AV block is generally more sinister than the Type I block and is usually indicative of a serious organic lesion in the conductive pathway below the AV node.

The atrial rate is regular with a constant PR interval, except when dropped beats occur due to conduction blockage in the bundle of His or in the bundle branches. The QRS pattern will be normal if the conduction block is in the bundle of His, and spread out if the block is situated in the left or right bundle branch (Fig. 2.86).

Third degree heart block

In third degree heart block there is a complete conduction block between the atria and the ventricles. Consequently, each set of chambers contracts at its own intrinsic rate and the P waves and the QRS complexes are completely dissociated. The intrinsic ventricular rate is slow (35–55/min) (Fig. 2.87).

Ectopic Beats

Ectopic foci may arise in either the atria or the ventricles, giving rise to premature contraction in the relevant chambers.

Premature atrial complexes

A focus outside the sinoatrial (SA) node stimulates a premature atrial contraction. The rhythm is irregular.

The ectopic focus gives rise to an abnormally shaped P wave which occurs before the expected normal P wave. This abnormal wave may be "buried"

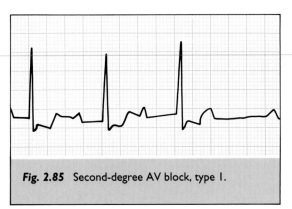

Fig. 2.85 Second-degree AV block, type I.

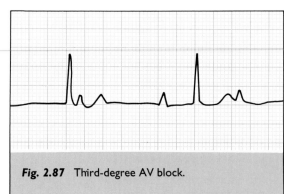

Fig. 2.87 Third-degree AV block.

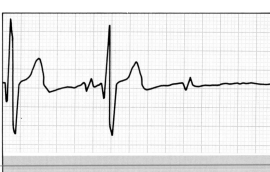

Fig. 2.86 Second-degree AV block, type 2.

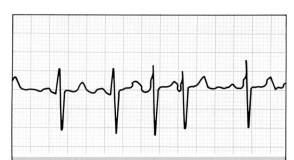

Fig. 2.88 Premature atrial complexes.

in the proceeding T wave. The QRS complex will be normal unless there is associated bundle branch block (Fig. 2.88).

Premature atrial complexes (PACs) are usually associated with stimulants such as caffeine or nicotine, exogenous or endogenous sympathometric agents, digitalis intoxication or hypoxia. Frequently no cause is apparent. No urgent therapy is required except to withdraw the cause.

Premature ventricular complexes

Premature ventricular complexes (PVCs) arise from an ectopic focus or foci within the ventricle causing premature ventricular contraction. Since the focus does not follow the normal conduction pathways, both ventricles do not contract simultaneously and the QRS complex is spread. The rate is irregular. The succeeding sinus P wave is usually buried within the normal QRS or following T wave.

Different ectopic focal sources will give rise to different shaped QRS complexes, and their degree of activity will be reflected in their frequency (Figs 2.89 & 2.90). The ectopic beat does not provide efficient cardiac ejection, so the urgency for treatment is related to the frequency of the PVCs. Treatment is discussed on p.73.

Atrial (Supraventricular) Tachycardia

Atrial tachycardia may be paroxysmal or non-paroxysmal. Non-paroxysmal tachycardia is usually associated with digitalis intoxication. Paroxysmal supraventricular tachycardia is more common; often the aetiology is obscure and benign, but it may be associated with valve disease, coronary atherosclerosis or hypoxia.

The atrial rate is regular and between 150 and 240/min. At rates below 200/min each P wave is usually followed by a QRS, but at higher rates a 2:1 block is likely to occur. The P waves may be buried within the preceding T wave. The QRS complexes are normal unless a bundle branch block has occurred as well (Fig. 2.91).

The management and treatment of paroxysmal atrial (supraventricular) tachycardia is shown in the algorithim on p.74.

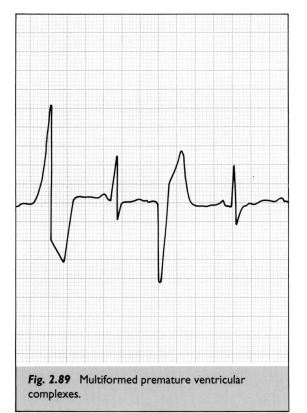

Fig. 2.89 Multiformed premature ventricular complexes.

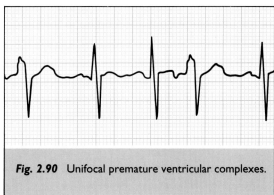

Fig. 2.90 Unifocal premature ventricular complexes.

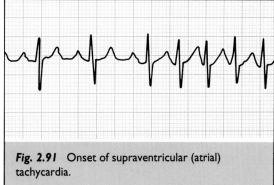

Fig. 2.91 Onset of supraventricular (atrial) tachycardia.

DEFIBRILLATION

Electrical defibrillation is the most effective method of converting ventricular fibrillation to a rhythm which generates a spontaneous cardiac output. It must, however, be applied early for success. A very substantial proportion of patients with witnessed arrest due to primary VF can be resuscitated if defibrillation is applied within the first one or two minutes. After four minutes the success rate drops exponentially as metabolic acidosis and other effects of hypoxia build up in the myocardium.

The urgency of early defibrillation in VF cannot be stressed too strongly.

Mode of Action

In VF the myocardial fibres are contracting in a disorganized haphazard fashion. The application of an electric shock to the heart has the effect of stimulating all myocardial fibres at the same instant, after which they lie dormant for a refractory period awaiting the next spontaneous stimulus arriving through the heart's conducting tissue. They then respond to this stimulus simultaneously in the normal fashion to produce a coordinated cardiac contraction.

Energy requirements

The output of a modern defibrillator is calibrated for "delivered energy", which is some 10 per cent less than the energy stored in the capacitor of the apparatus because there is a loss down the wire between apparatus and the electrodes. The unit of energy for defibrillators is the Joule (J = Watt/second).

Certain low energy levels do not reach the threshold required for ventricular defibrillation, moderate levels have a high probability of successful conversion, but higher levels do not necessarily achieve better success rates and may cause cardiac muscle damage. Optimum energy levels for external defibrillation through the chest wall may be calculated on a body weight basis (Fig. 2.92). It has been shown that best benefits for an adult of 70kg come from an initial shock of 200J, but higher energy shocks are not required initially for adults of greater weight.

It is generally agreed that the first two shocks should be of the same energy, and that the third and subsequent shocks should be approximately twice

this level. Thus for adults the sequence should be:
- Initial shock — 200J.
- Second shock — 200J.
- Third (and subsequent) shocks — 360J.

The maximum energy output delivered by most defibrillators is 360J, representing 400J stored energy.

Energy requirements for external defibrillation

When the defibrillator paddles are applied directly to the heart the energy requirements are considerably less because of the absence of transthoracic impedance. As a rough guide, the energy requirements are 10 per cent of those needed for external defibrillation (see Fig. 2.92).

Defibrillators

Defibrillators deliver a variable high-voltage DC shock. The power source may be derived either from a rechargeable battery or from an AC mains supply which is converted to DC and stored in a capacitor. Some models offer both a mains supply and a rechargeable battery. These are most suitable for hospital use. Battery-only models are suitable for prehospital care. Defibrillators may be of three types:
- Manual.
- Semi-automatic.
- Automatic.

Fig. 2.92 Energy requirements for initial defibrillaton shocks in ventricular fibrillation.

Body weight (kg)	Energy requirements (J)
≥70	200
50	100
25	50
10	20
Other weights 2J/kg	

Manually operated defibrillators

Modern defibrillators incorporate an ECG oscilloscope which enables the ECG to be monitored directly from the paddle electrodes. They also include a socket and three-lead flex for attachment to standard pre-gelled adhesive monitoring chest electrodes. Some models allow the ECG and defibrillator to be separated if required.

The defibrillator paddle electrodes should be 10cm in diameter for adults, reducing to 8cm for larger children and 4.5cm for infants. For internal defibrillation the paddle size should range from 6cm for adults to 2cm for infants. Facilities for internal defibrillation should be incorporated in defibrillators planned for use in areas where open chest cardiac compression may be used, for example operating rooms and emergency departments.

Many modern defibrillators are equipped with silicon chip technology and incorporate pre-use checks, and record rhythm, performance and other relevant data such as time, date and patient thoracic

impedance. All machines incorporate the following operating controls (Fig. 2.93):
- Power on/off switch.
- Select energy dial.
- Charge button.
- Discharge buttons.
- Recording switch (optional).

In addition, some models incorporate a synchronize selector switch which synchronizes delivery of the shock with the peak of the R wave of the ECG. The synchronized mode is used in cardioversion of ventricular tachycardia or atrial fibrillation.

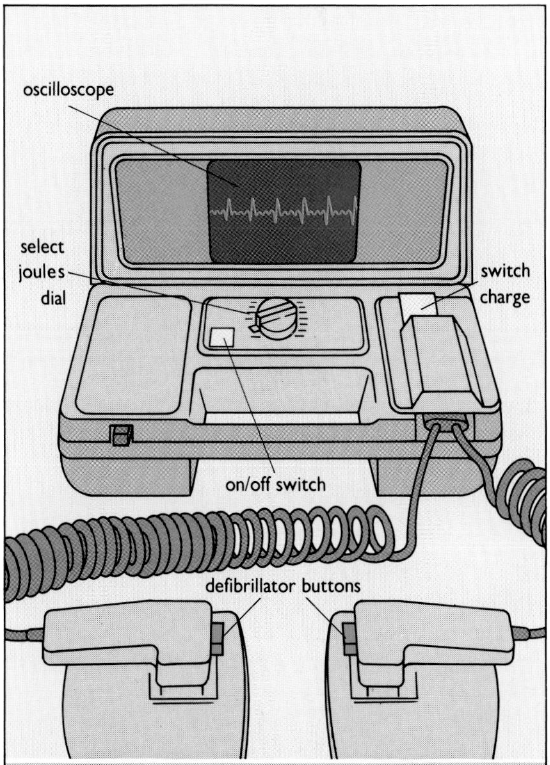

The synchronized mode should not be used in VF as there is no R wave and delivery of the shock will be delayed indefinitely.

Technique of manual defibrillation of VF
1 Remove paddle electrodes from locating slots.
2 Turn power on.
3 Discontinue chest compressions and ventilation.
4 Apply one paddle electrode firmly (using a pressure equivalent to 10kg weight) over the apex of the heart and the other along the right sternal border just beneath the clavicle (see Fig. 2.74).
5 Observe ECG (check for artefacts).
6 Remove paddle electrodes.
7 Continue chest compressions and ventilation.
8 Apply defibrillator contact pads to the chest over the apex and sternal positions, or apply electrode jelly to the paddle surfaces to prepare them for use.
9 Adjust energy select dial to the appropriate level for the patient (200J for adult).
10 Press charge.
11 Order the rescuers to stand back and not to touch the patient.

The defibrillator is potentially dangerous to personnel around the patient. Always issue a clear order to stand back prior to discharging the shock.

Fig. 2.93 Controls for an ECG defibrillator.

12 Press defibrillate button on both electrodes ......

57

...... to discharge shock (the patient will jactitate if a shock has been discharged).

13 Continue chest compressions and ventilation for 15 seconds (to allow ECG oscilloscope to recover).

14 Feel for carotid pulse and check ECG.

15 Repeat process if VF persists.

Defibrillator contact pads are much superior to electrode jelly which tends to get smeared over the entire chest wall by chest compressions. Defibrillation then results in the shock passing superficially around the chest wall surface which produces a frightening arc flashing between the electrodes, surface burning of the patient's chest and failure to defibrillate the heart. Always ensure that there is a gap in the jelly spread between the two electrodes.

---

16 Always ensure that the patient's chest is dry (for example, victims of near drowning), otherwise similar problems may occur.

Semi-automatic defibrillator

Semi-automatic defibrillators use computer technology to interpret the ECG from large 10cm adhesive electrodes and offer advice as to whether defibrillation is appropriate. If defibrillation is required, the operator presses the defibrillate button on the apparatus and a predetermined (adult) shock is delivered through the larger adhesive electrodes. A verbal warning that defibrillation is going to occur is given by the machine itself.

This type of machine has the advantages that artefacts are minimized by the use of large adhesive electrodes and that the ECG interpretation is made automatically and does not require a trained operator. The ultimate decision to defibrillate does, however, rest with the operator. The ECG is displayed on an oscilloscope, which is better than the pulse bar graph used in some earlier models. The technology allows sophisticated recording and play-back systems which are valuable in teaching and audit (Fig. 2.94).

Semi-automatic defibrillators are most suitable for use by the ambulance service and in hospital areas where cardiac arrests are rare and staff are relatively inexperienced. The minor drawback of the semi-automatic devices is that they are relatively inflexible and deliver predetermined shock energy levels for adults (according to the guidelines of the American Heart Association, the Resuscitation Council UK and the European and Australian Resuscitation Councils). For children, in whom VF is very rare anyway, they are therefore not suitable without modification. Some models incorporate an override facility using a cassette which can be issued to specially trained personnel. This increases the flexibility and versatility of the performance. Suitable models include the Laerdal Heartstart 3000, and the Physio Control 300 with ECG attachment, and the Marquette Semi-Automatic defibrillator.

Technique of semi-automatic defibrillation of VF

1 Apply the adhesive electrodes to the apex and sternal positions (see Fig. 2.74).

2 Turn on the apparatus.

3 Observe the ECG trace.

4 Read the instructions on the VDU.

5 Press the defibrillate button if indicated.

6 Listen to the audible warnings issued by the apparatus.

7 Stand back.

8 Observe delivery of shock.

9 Check for carotid pulse.

10 Observe VDU for ECG interpretation and further instructions.

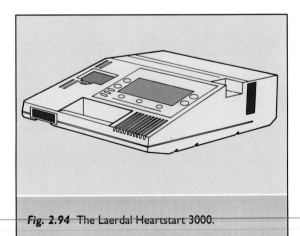

Fig. 2.94 The Laerdal Heartstart 3000.

Automatic defibrillators

Automatic defibrillators work on the same principle as the semi-automatic type except that the apparatus (after delivering an audible warning) delivers the shock to the patient in VF without any further action by the operator. They are designed for use by relatively unskilled lay personnel, for example relatives of at-risk patients, airline cabin crew, railway staff, firemen, first aid personnel, etc.

The only action required by the rescuer, when faced with a victim who is unresponsive to basic life support measures, is to apply the large adhesive electrodes in the apex and sternum positions and turn on the apparatus. The appropriate action for treating VF by defibrillation will follow.

EMERGENCY CARDIAC PACING

Emergency cardiac pacing is indicated in patients with:
- Severe bradycardia unresponsive to atropine or isoprenaline.
- Witnessed asystole with persistent P waves unresponsive to adrenaline, atropine or other stimulants, where the prognosis is not thought to be hopeless.

The hypoxic acidotic heart will not respond to pacing. Emergency pacing of the heart can be accomplished by the following techniques:
- External fist pacing (see p.44).
- Transcutaneous thoracic electrical pacing.
- Transvenous electrical pacing.

Transcutaneous thoracic pacing

Transcutaneous thoracic electrical pacing technology has improved to reduce painful voluntary chest muscle contractions. Stimuli of 25–150V lasting 2–3 milliseconds are delivered at a rate of 70/min via large adhesive electrodes applied to the apex and sternum positions.

Some defibrillators incorporate a transcutaneous thoracic pacing facility.

Transvenous pacing

Transvenous electrical pacing is accomplished by a bipolar catheter inserted via the internal jugular, subclavian, brachial or femoral vein into the right atrium or ventricle under ECG guidance. Once in a satisfactory position the catheter is connected to a standard pacing box.

DRUG THERAPY

Primary Agents

In cardiac arrest three first-line drugs should be immediately to hand. These are:
- Adrenaline (epinephrine).
- Lignocaine (lidocaine).
- Atropine.

Adrenaline (epinephrine)

Adrenaline is a catecholamine with both α and β effects. It has a complex effect on the cardiovascular system because some of the original actions are modified by reflex activity. Its main actions include:
- Increase in systemic vascular resistance.
- Increase in systolic and diastolic arterial pressure.
- Increase in myocardial contractility and automaticity.
- Increase in heart rate.

As a result it improves cerebral and coronary perfusion and stimulates the failing myocardium directly. The improvement in cerebral and coronary perfusion is probably the principal beneficial effect in cardiac arrest. No other cardiovascular stimulant has yet been found to rival adrenaline in clinical practice.

■ INDICATIONS
Adrenaline is indicated in the following instances:
- Asystole.
- Electromechanical dissociation.
- Fading fine VF.
- Refractory cardiogenic shock in selected patients, for example post-cardiopulmonary bypass.

■ DOSAGE
Adrenaline is given intravenously in an initial dose of 10ml of 1/10,000 solution (1mg) in adults. This dose can be repeated almost immediately if the desired effect is not achieved. Further doses may be given but hopes fade if the initial response is not encouraging. The dose in children is $100\mu g/kg$.

Lignocaine (lidocaine)

Lignocaine suppresses ventricular arrhythmias and ectopic foci. Its main actions include:
- Reduction of automaticity.
- Depression of conduction in resistant pathways.
- Reduction of fibrillation potential and recurrence.
- Depression of myocardial contractility and arterial blood pressure (in larger doses).

■ INDICATIONS

Lignocaine is indicated in the following instances:

- Persistent coarse VF.
- Ventricular tachycardia.
- PVCs in patients with accompanying hypotension due to ischaemic heart disease.
- PVCs which are close-coupled, multiform or occurring with a frequency greater than 1:6.

■ DOSAGE

Lignocaine is given slowly over a period of 2 minutes in a dose of 1mg/kg. Additional bolus doses of 0.5mg/kg can be given every 5–10 minutes, progressing to an infusion of 30–500μg/kg/min (2–4mg/min in an adult) to achieve and retain myocardial stability but reducing after two hours.

Atropine

Atropine opposes parasympathetic activity. It is used in cardiac arrest for its vagolytic effect to counter intense vagal activity which may have been the original cause of asystole, or to prevent arrest following bradycardia with hypotension.

■ INDICATIONS

Atropine is indicated in the following instances:

- Asystole (after adrenaline has failed).
- Sinus bradycardia with hypotension (atropine is not indicated if the bradycardia is not associated with cardiovascular compromise).
- Heart block of all types (rarely effective).
- To counter overdoses of parasympathetic agents, for example neostigmine, physostigmine and toxic nerve agents.

■ DOSAGE

Atropine is given in a dose of 1–3mg in adults. Much larger doses may be needed in nerve agent intoxication.

Secondary Agents

Secondary agents may be required to support the action of the primary drugs after cardiac arrest has been converted to a spontaneous rhythm (Fig. 2.95).

Adrenergic agents

■ **ISOPRENALINE (ISOPROTERENOL)**

Isoprenaline has, almost exclusively, β-adrenergic effects only.

■ INDICATIONS

It is used in heart block of all types and in sinus tachycardia with hypotension refractory to atropine therapy.

■ DOSAGE

Isoprenaline is usually administered as an intravenous infusion at a rate of 0.02–0.04μg/kg/min — 2–10μg/min in an adult.

■ **NORADRENALINE (NOREPINEPHRINE)**

Noradrenaline is a potent α-adrenergic agent with additional β effects, particularly at higher dose levels. The drug is not used in the immediate cardiac arrest situation because its profound vasoconstriction action in such conditions leads to tissue underperfusion and acidosis, and its β action increases myocardial oxygen requirements.

adrenergic agents	antiarrhythmic agents	agents countering metabolic acidosis	miscellaneous agents
isoprenaline (isoproterenol) noradrenaline (norepinephrine) dopamine dobutamine	bretylium verapamil amiodarone beta-blocking agents, e.g. propranolol or labetalol	sodium bicarbonate carbicarb	calcium chloride or gluconate nitroglycerine frusemide (furosemide)

Fig. 2.95 Secondary agents supporting the action of primary drugs in cardiac arrest.

■ INDICATIONS

It is used in refractory cardiogenic shock to maintain an adequate perfusion pressure temporarily while the underlying pathological processes are dealt with.

■ DOSAGE

Noradrenaline is given by i.v. infusion of a diluted solution titrated just to control the arterial pressure at a reasonable level. In an adult, $2\mu g/min$ is generally used as a starting dose.

> Noradrenaline should only be administered by a long central i.v. line. Administration into a peripheral vein will quickly cause local phlebitis and thrombosis, and extravasation will cause necrosis of the adjacent tissues.

■ DOPAMINE

Dopamine has both α– and β_2–adrenergic actions. The α activity is more marked at higher dose rates and may be counterproductive, as the associated increase in myocardial oxygen requirement may exceed the myocardial blood flow.

■ INDICATIONS

Dopamine is not used in the immediate cardiac arrest situation but may be valuable to support cardiac and renal output in the post-arrest phase.

■ DOSAGE

Dopamine is given by i.v. infusion. An amount of the drug in milligrams equal to six times the patient's body weight in kilograms is made up to 50ml. With this mixture, the flow rate in ml/h is equal to the $\mu g/kg/h$ of the drug given to the patient.

■ DOBUTAMINE

Dobutamine has a complex adrenergic action stimulating β_1, β_2 and α receptors. The net result is that cardiac output is increased and there is a modest vasodilator effect as the β_2 activity is greater than the α activity.

■ INDICATIONS

Dobutamine is not used in the immediate cardiac arrest situation but may be of value in sustaining tissue perfusion in the post-arrest period.

■ DOSAGE

Dobutamine is also given by i.v. infusion at the rate of $2.5–10.0\mu g/kg/min$ in adults.

Antiarrhythmic agents

■ **BRETYLIUM TOSYLATE**

Bretylium has a complex pharmacological action, first stimulating adrenergic receptors and then causing adrenergic blockade. It decreases the defibrillation potential and also reduces the likelihood of recurrence of ventricular fibrillation or ventricular tachycardia.

■ INDICATIONS

Bretylium is used in VF or VT when lignocaine in combination with defibrillation has failed, and in refractory cases of ventricular ectopy.

■ DOSAGE

5mg/kg is given i.v., repeated two or three times if necessary.

■ **VERAPAMIL**

Verapamil is a calcium-blocking agent which reduces myocardial oxygen consumption. It is a negative inotrope which protects the myocardium but which may reduce cardiac output. It slows conduction through the AV node and therefore is particularly useful in tachycardia and re-entrant dysrhythmias.

■ INDICATIONS

Verapamil is used in paroxysmal supraventricular tachycardia. It is not used in cardiac arrest nor in ventricular tachycardia because of its negative inotropic action.

■ DOSAGE

0.075–0.15mg/kg as a bolus, repeated as necessary up to a total of 10mg in an adult.

■ **AMIODARONE**

Amioderone is a class III antiarrhythmic agent which prolongs the refractory period without altering the resting membrane potential or rate of depolarization. The re-excitation interval is prolonged and hence arrhythmias are suppressed. Potentially the fibrillation threshold is elevated but the drug has not yet been proven in the management of VF or VT.

■ INDICATIONS

Amiodarone is indicated in ventricular ectopy when hypotension is present. It may also be used in refractory VF or VT unresponsive to lignocaine.

■ DOSAGE

2.5–10.0mg/kg by i.v. injection.

■ **BETA-BLOCKING AGENTS**

Beta-blocking agents prevent catecholamines from binding to their receptors. They therefore reduce heart rate, arterial pressure and myocardial oxygen requirements. However, they do also reduce myocardial contractility and thus have no place during cardiac arrest.

■ INDICATIONS

Control of recurrent VF or VT when other measures have failed and the cause is related to excessive β-adrenergic stimulation.

■ DOSAGE

Propranolol should be given to adults in a dose of 5–10mg slowly by i.v. over 5 minutes. Labetalol is an alternative agent, given in a dose of 5mg for an adult, followed by an infusion of 15–20mg/h.

Agents countering metabolic acidosis

■ SODIUM BICARBONATE

Sodium bicarbonate has been traditionally used to combat the metabolic acidosis that inevitably follows a moderately prolonged period of cardiac arrest. However, it is now realized that previous protocols dictated that too much was given too early, and recent recommendations from the American Heart Association and the Resuscitation Councils, both in the UK and Australia, advise that the drug should not be given before 20 minutes of arrest has elapsed and then only in modest dosage. It has been pointed out that much of the acidosis can be controlled by satisfactory artificial ventilation, and that hypernatraemia and metabolic alkalosis may occur with excessive bicarbonate administration.

■ DOSAGE

Sodium bicarbonate is given "blindly" in a single dose of 1mEq/kg after 20 minutes of arrest. Further administration should be guided by arterial pH and blood gas analysis. As a guide the total dose of bicarbonate required should be calculated as follows:

$$\text{sodium bicarbonate (mEq)} = \frac{\text{Base deficit (mEq)} \times \text{body weight(kg)}}{4}$$

Half of this dose should be given initially and further increments should be guided by more estimations of the base deficit. A base deficit of 5mEq is acceptable.

Sodium bicarbonate is extremely irritant and venous extravasation is usually followed by skin necrosis. It should always be given through a central intravenous line.

■ **CARBICARB**

Carbicarb is a new agent which is designed to replace bicarbonate and is claimed to reduce the incidence of hyponatraemia and hyperosmolality experienced with bicarbonate. Further evaluation is required before its widespread introduction into clinical practice.

Miscellaneous agents

■ **CALCIUM IONS**

Calcium ions increase myocardial contractility but also increase coronary artery tonus and excitability, limiting the value of calcium in cardiac arrest due to primary cardiac causes, except after bypass surgery. The ions are available as either calcium chloride (10%) or calcium gluconate (10%).

■ INDICATIONS

Calcium is only indicated in cases of asystole or EMD due to nonprimary cardiac causes when adrenaline has failed.

■ DOSAGE   Calcium chloride (10%) is given in an i.v. dose of 2–4mg/kg (approximately 5ml of 10% solution). Calcium gluconate (10%) contains less ionized calcium and therefore the dose should be doubled.

■ **NITROGLYCERIN**   Nitroglycerin acts as an arterial and venous vasodilator reducing the cardiac preload and afterload. It also directly improves the coronary artery blood flow.

■ INDICATIONS

Nitroglycerin has no place in the immediate management of cardiac arrest but is indicated in the post-arrest phase to control hypertension and reduce myocardial ischaemia.

■ DOSAGE

Nitroglycerin is given by i.v. infusion in a dose of 2–10μg/kg/h in adults.

■ **FRUSEMIDE (FUROSEMIDE)**

Frusemide is a diuretic acting by inhibiting sodium reabsorption in the loop of Henle.

■ INDICATIONS

Frusemide is indicated in the post-arrest phase if overload cardiac failure and pulmonary oedema are present.

■ DOSAGE

Frusemide is given in an intravenous dose of 0.5–1.0mg/kg. Diuresis occurs about 30 minutes after injection. The dose may be repeated after one hour if indicated.

> Potassium levels should be carefully monitored after the administration of frusemide.

Routes of Administration for Drugs in Cardiac Arrest

Four routes are available for the administration of certain drugs in cardiopulmonary resuscitation:
- Intravenous.
- Endobronchial.
- Intracardiac.
- Intraosseous.

The intravenous route

All drugs may be given by this route but during cardiac arrest a 14–16G central line (internal or external jugular, or subclavian or long line from the antecubital fossa; see Section 3) must be used because circulation through the peripheral veins is minimal during external chest compressions. Irritant agents such as sodium bicarbonate, noradrenaline and calcium chloride must always be given by a central line.

The endobronchial route

Atropine and lignocaine may also be given endobronchially using a nebulizing endpiece fitted to the syringe for injection down the endotracheal tube. Adrenaline may also be given by this route, although local vasoconstriction in the lungs may reduce uptake. The dose for all of these drugs given by the endobronchial route is twice the intravenous dose. A volume of 10ml should be used.

> The endobronchial route is *not* suitable for sodium bicarbonate or calcium ions and has not been assessed for other agents. Its use should therefore be reserved for atropine, lignocaine and adrenaline.

The intracardiac route

This route can be used in open-chest CPR for a variety of drugs, but during closed-chest CPR it should only be considered as a last resort if it proves impossible to establish an intravenous or endotracheal route.

Blind intracardiac injections may damage a coronary artery, lodge in the myocardium rather than the chamber, or cause a pneumothorax or cardiac tamponade. Only adrenaline should be given blindly by this route.

> **Technique**
> 1 The paraxiphoid approach is safest (Fig. 2.96).
> 2 Introduce a long 22G needle below the ribcage, one finger-breadth to the left of the xiphoid process.
> 3 Advance the needle cephelad, posteriorly and laterally, for about 6–10cm, aspirating at frequent intervals until a free flow of blood appears in the syringe.
> 4 The intracardiac dose of adrenaline is 10ml of 1/10,000 solution.

The intraosseous route

This route may be useful in children where venous access is difficult.

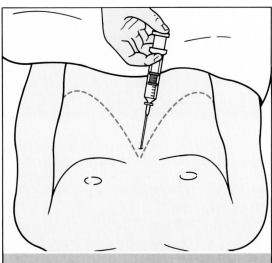

Fig. 2.96 The paraxiphoid approach for intracardiac injections.

Presentation of Drugs Used in CPR

Drugs used in the immediate resuscitation phase (adrenaline, atropine, lignocaine, bicarbonate, isoprenaline, calcium chloride, etc.) are available in preloaded syringes containing the usual adult dose in a convenient concentration (International Medical Systems Ltd). This system has very considerable advantages of speed and convenience over conventional ampoules, syringes and needles.

The equipment consists of a syringe barrel with a central needle which pierces the bung of a vial containing the drug (Fig. 2.97). This central needle is contiguous with the needle or Luer fitting emitting from the syringe barrel.

Technique

1 Remove the syringe barrel and vial from the container.
2 Push off the covers from the syringe barrel and vial.
3 Screw the barrel and vial together.
4 Eject air from the central needle until fluid flows from the external needle.
5 Either (i) inject the drug via a resealable port into an i.v. giving set, or (ii) break off the external part of the needle to leave a male Luer fitting for injection into a female Luer fitting in the i.v. cannula or three-way tap (alternatively this fitting may be attached to a nebulizer fitment for endobronchial use).
6 Do not use the needle of the preloaded syringe for direct venepuncture as it cannot be removed from the syringe

Thrombolytic Therapy

The early use of thrombolytic therapy using agents such as streptokinase with aspirin as an adjuvant improves mortality substantially in patients with myocardial infarction. The main contraindications to this therapy are associated with an increased risk of haemorrhage due to anticoagulant therapy or platelet deficiency or from potential sources of bleeding such as gastrointestinal and urinary tract ulceration, recent obstetric delivery or wounding. External chest compressions may cause rib fractures or soft tissue injury, which are a potential source of bleeding, and, therefore, they represent a relative contraindication to thrombolytic therapy if carried out with force over a period of more than a few minutes. The details of thrombolytic therapy are outside the scope of this book

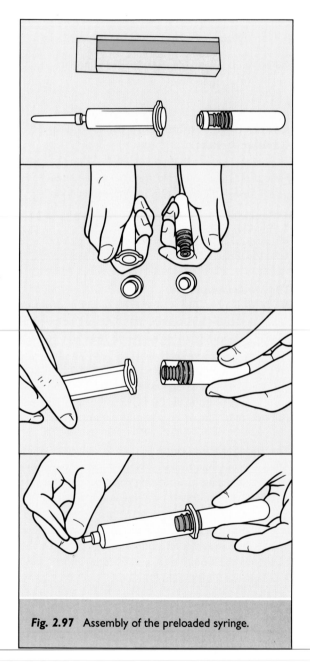

Fig. 2.97 Assembly of the preloaded syringe.

RESUSCITATION ALGORITHMS

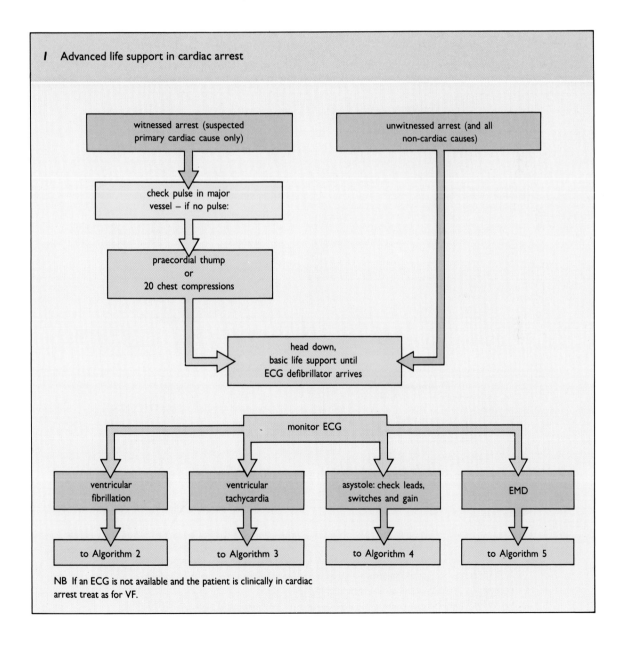

1 Advanced life support in cardiac arrest

witnessed arrest (suspected
primary cardiac cause only)

unwitnessed arrest (and all
non-cardiac causes)

check pulse in major
vessel – if no pulse:

praecordial thump
or
20 chest compressions

head down,
basic life support until
ECG defibrillator arrives

monitor ECG

ventricular fibrillation	ventricular tachycardia	asystole: check leads, switches and gain	EMD
to Algorithm 2	to Algorithm 3	to Algorithm 4	to Algorithm 5

NB If an ECG is not available and the patient is clinically in cardiac
arrest treat as for VF.

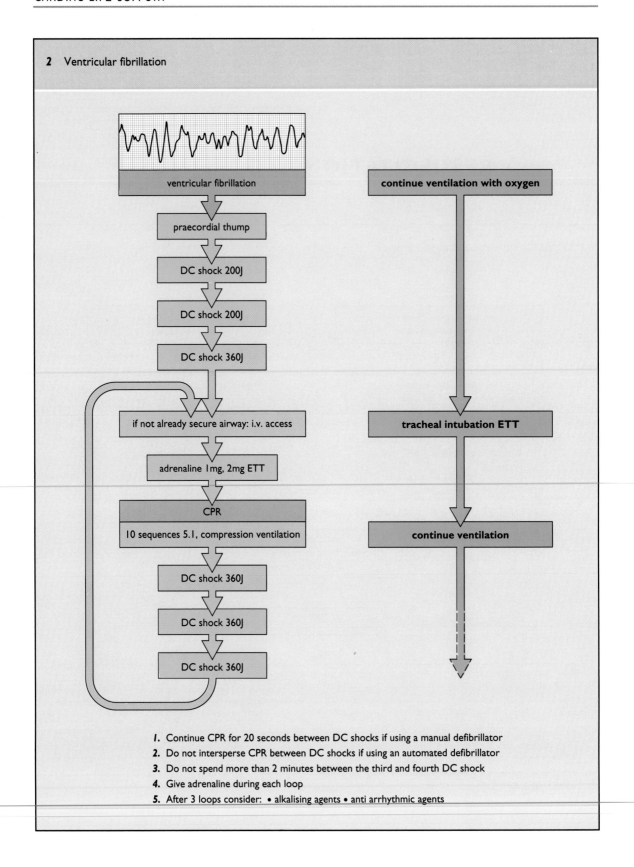

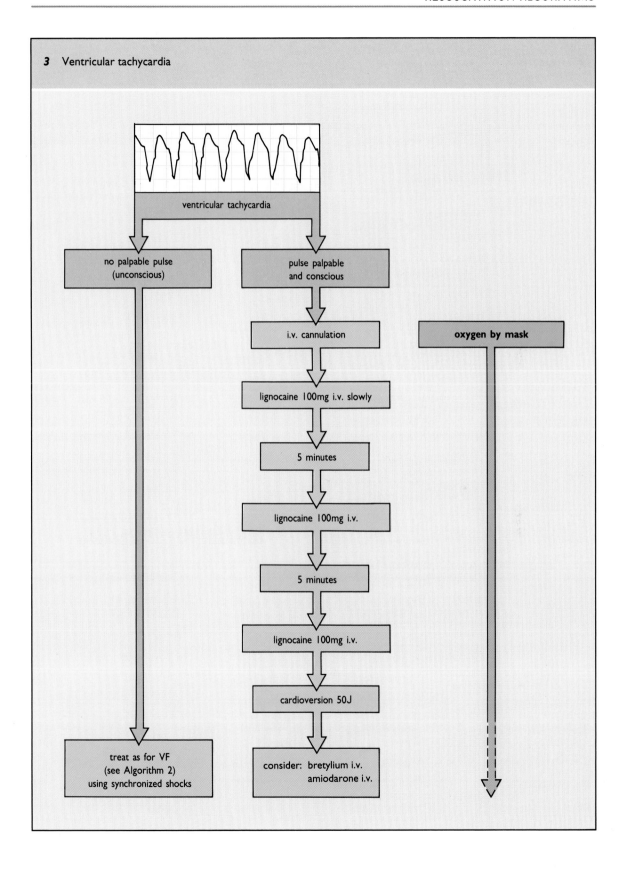

3 Ventricular tachycardia

ventricular tachycardia

no palpable pulse
(unconscious)

pulse palpable
and conscious

i.v. cannulation

lignocaine 100mg i.v. slowly

5 minutes

lignocaine 100mg i.v.

5 minutes

lignocaine 100mg i.v.

cardioversion 50J

oxygen by mask

treat as for VF
(see Algorithm 2)
using synchronized shocks

consider: bretylium i.v.
amiodarone i.v.

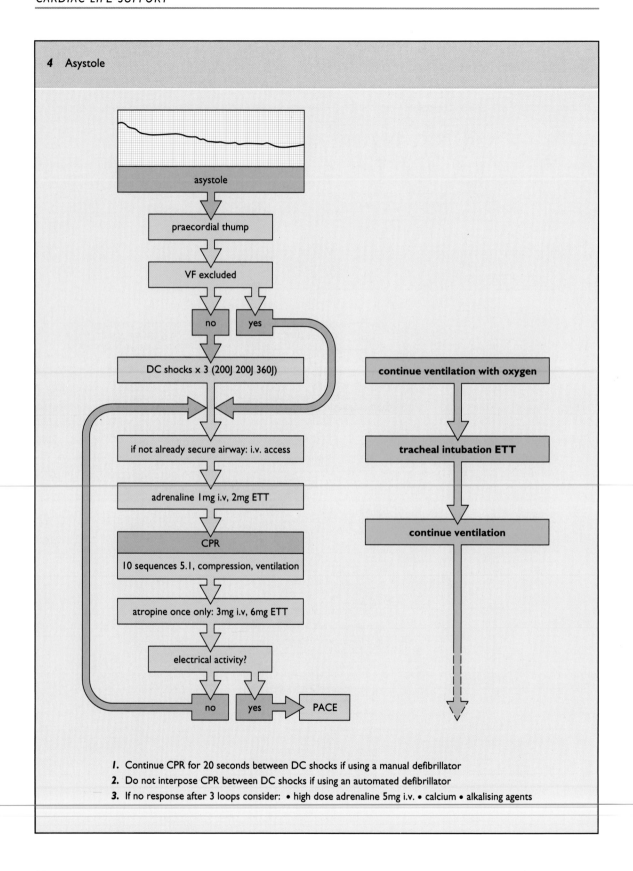

4 Asystole

asystole

praecordial thump

VF excluded

no   yes

DC shocks x 3 (200J 200J 360J)

if not already secure airway: i.v. access

adrenaline 1mg i.v, 2mg ETT

CPR

10 sequences 5.1, compression, ventilation

atropine once only: 3mg i.v, 6mg ETT

electrical activity?

no   yes   PACE

continue ventilation with oxygen

tracheal intubation ETT

continue ventilation

1. Continue CPR for 20 seconds between DC shocks if using a manual defibrillator

2. Do not interpose CPR between DC shocks if using an automated defibrillator

3. If no response after 3 loops consider: • high dose adrenaline 5mg i.v. • calcium • alkalising agents

5 Electromechanical dissociation (EMD)

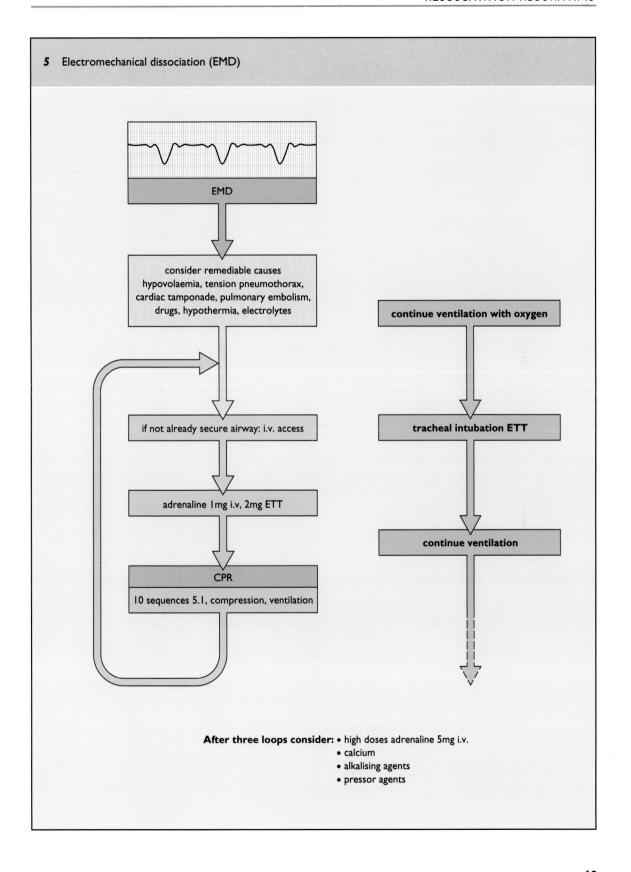

EMD

consider remediable causes
hypovolaemia, tension pneumothorax,
cardiac tamponade, pulmonary embolism,
drugs, hypothermia, electrolytes

continue ventilation with oxygen

if not already secure airway: i.v. access

tracheal intubation ETT

adrenaline 1mg i.v, 2mg ETT

continue ventilation

CPR

10 sequences 5.1, compression, ventilation

After three loops consider: • high doses adrenaline 5mg i.v.
• calcium
• alkalising agents
• pressor agents

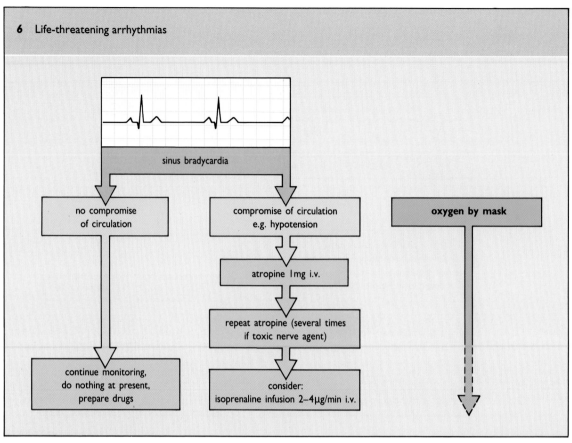

6 Life-threatening arrhythmias

sinus bradycardia

no compromise
of circulation

compromise of circulation
e.g. hypotension

oxygen by mask

atropine 1mg i.v.

repeat atropine (several times
if toxic nerve agent)

continue monitoring,
do nothing at present,
prepare drugs

consider:
isoprenaline infusion 2–4µg/min i.v.

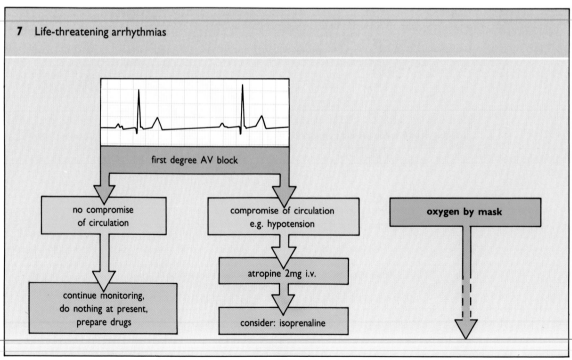

7 Life-threatening arrhythmias

first degree AV block

no compromise
of circulation

compromise of circulation
e.g. hypotension

oxygen by mask

atropine 2mg i.v.

continue monitoring,
do nothing at present,
prepare drugs

consider: isoprenaline

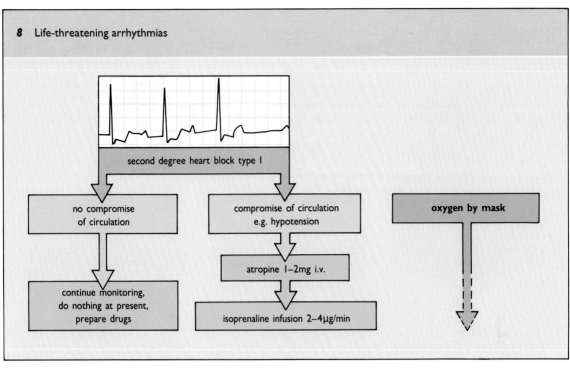

8 Life-threatening arrhythmias

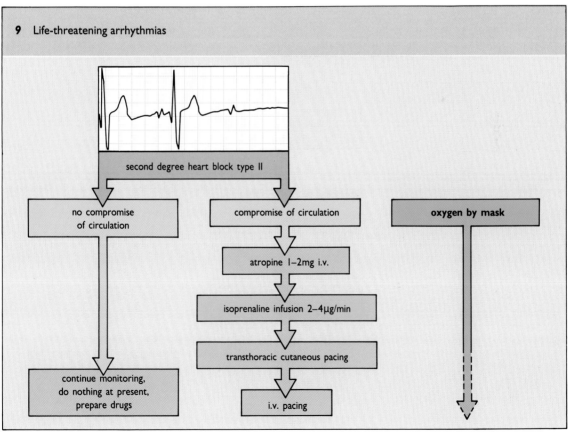

9 Life-threatening arrhythmias

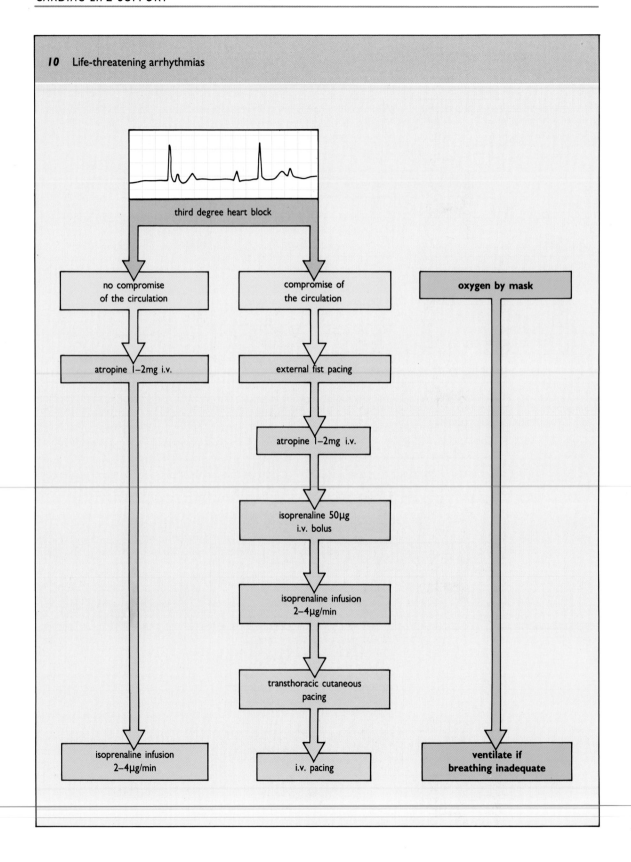

10 Life-threatening arrhythmias

third degree heart block

| no compromise of the circulation | compromise of the circulation | **oxygen by mask** |

atropine 1–2mg i.v.

external fist pacing

atropine 1–2mg i.v.

isoprenaline 50μg i.v. bolus

isoprenaline infusion 2–4μg/min

transthoracic cutaneous pacing

isoprenaline infusion 2–4μg/min

i.v. pacing

ventilate if breathing inadequate

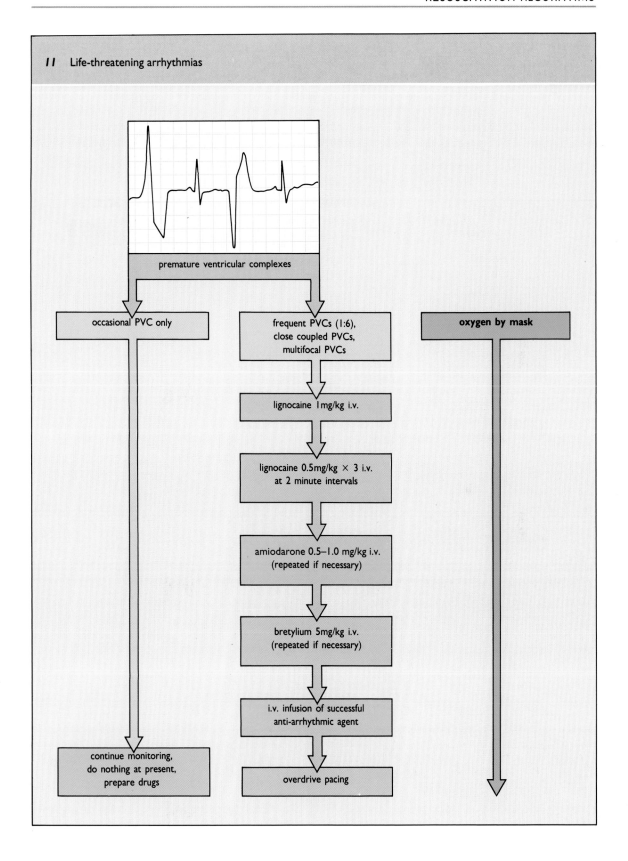

11   Life-threatening arrhythmias

premature ventricular complexes

occasional PVC only

frequent PVCs (1:6), close coupled PVCs, multifocal PVCs

oxygen by mask

lignocaine 1mg/kg i.v.

lignocaine 0.5mg/kg × 3 i.v. at 2 minute intervals

amiodarone 0.5–1.0 mg/kg i.v. (repeated if necessary)

bretylium 5mg/kg i.v. (repeated if necessary)

i.v. infusion of successful anti-arrhythmic agent

continue monitoring, do nothing at present, prepare drugs

overdrive pacing

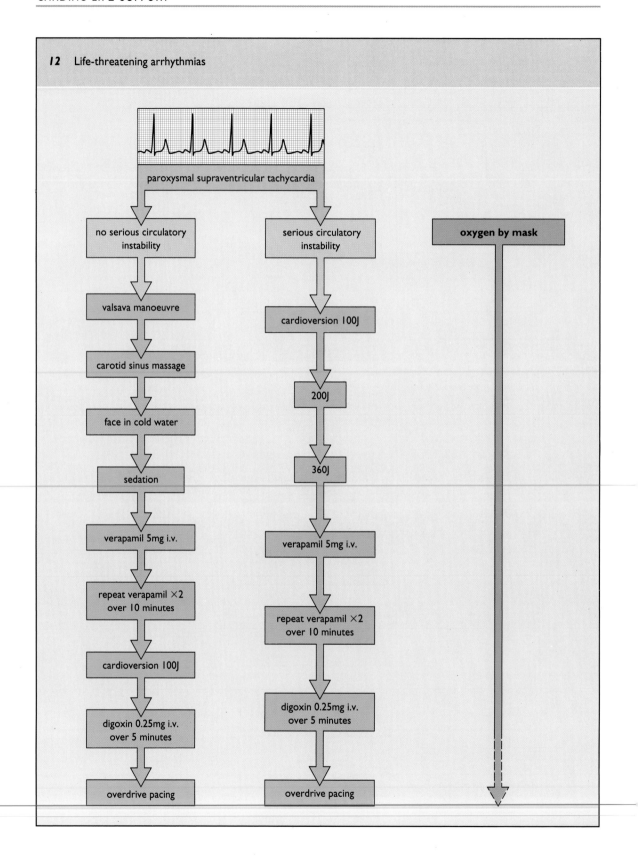

12   Life-threatening arrhythmias

paroxysmal supraventricular tachycardia

| no serious circulatory instability | serious circulatory instability | **oxygen by mask** |

no serious circulatory instability → valsava manoeuvre → carotid sinus massage → face in cold water → sedation → verapamil 5mg i.v. → repeat verapamil ×2 over 10 minutes → cardioversion 100J → digoxin 0.25mg i.v. over 5 minutes → overdrive pacing

serious circulatory instability → cardioversion 100J → 200J → 360J → verapamil 5mg i.v. → repeat verapamil ×2 over 10 minutes → digoxin 0.25mg i.v. over 5 minutes → overdrive pacing

TRAUMA LIFE SUPPORT

PRINCIPLES, INITIAL ASSESSMENT AND IMMEDIATE MANAGEMENT

Principles

Resuscitation after trauma broadly follows the same immediate life support principles as resuscitation after primary cardiac insufficiency or arrest, with emphasis being placed on a rapid initial assessment followed by immediate restoration of the vital functions of the airway, breathing and the circulation as required.

Many of the techniques for support of vital functions are common to both cardiac and trauma life support. However, there are procedures which are more specifically relevant to the primary cause. Thus cardiac resuscitation places particular emphasis on early defibrillation and drug therapy, while resuscitation after major trauma requires treatment of hypovolaemia and may need surgical control of haemorrhage and repair or resection of injured tissues.

This section will deal with the overall management of the seriously injured patient, referring as appropriate to certain techniques already covered in Section 2.

Initial assessment and immediate management

The vital functions of the critically injured patient must be rapidly assessed. The evaluation should follow an orderly sequence, to ensure that the correct priorities are met and that less obvious injuries are not overlooked, along the following lines:
- Primary Survey
- Resuscitation of vital functions
- Secondary Survey
- Definitive care

THE PRIMARY SURVEY

The Primary Survey is designed to identify life-threatening injuries from the history of the incident and from an examination of the airway, breathing and the circulation.

If serious impairment of any of these vital functions is apparent treatment should be instigated immediately. History-taking can run concurrently with this rapid examination. The pattern of examination and history-taking is detailed in Figure 3.1. The survey should be rapid, and life-threatening conditions such as airway obstruction, inadequate ventilation and profound hypovolaemia should be corrected as soon as they are discovered.

The vital functions examined in the Primary Survey should be continually reassessed.

All patients with multiple injuries or serious blunt trauma to the head and neck should be assumed to have a cervical spine injury and the head and neck should be held in a stable position while the airway is aligned and cleared (see p.15).

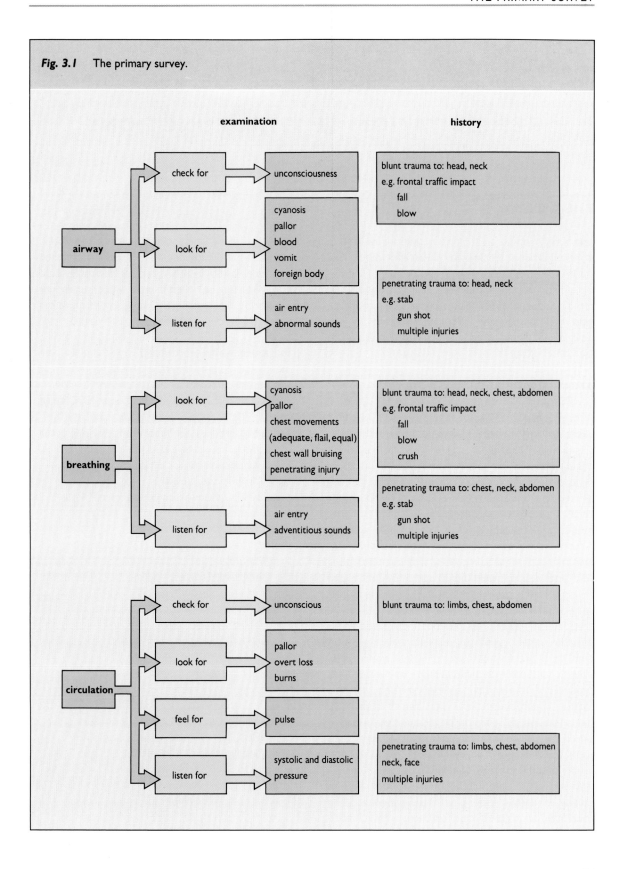

Fig. 3.1 The primary survey.

RESUSCITATION OF VITAL FUNCTIONS

THE AIRWAY

The airway should be aligned by cautious head neck positioning, chin lift and jaw thrust if required (see pp.15–16).

Foreign matter in the oropharynx should be removed under direct vision using a laryngoscope with suction through a Yankauer suction end for fluid material and Magill Forceps for solid objects (see pp.17-19).

Tracheal intubation in the injured

In many cases the airway patency can be maintained using an oro- or nasopharyngeal airway, but there remains the danger of gastric contents or blood being aspirated in unconscious patients. In these patients therefore tracheal intubation should be considered (see pp.26–28). However to accomplish tracheal intubation, unconsciousness must be profound. Attempts which result in a struggle with the patient cause positive harm and may result in laryngeal spasm, trauma, an increase in intracranial pressure and venous bleeding in the head and neck region. In such patients, when tracheal intubation is considered essential, a muscle relaxant should be used. Succinyl choline is commonly used because it provides rapid, profound relaxation with a short duration of action, but it may raise intracranial pressure in patients with head injuries and sometimes produces a bradycardia. Non-depolarizing relaxants such as vecuronium take a little longer to produce full relaxation and have a longer duration of action which may make for difficulty in elucidating certain signs, for example pain, tenderness, guarding, and rebound in the further examination of the patient.

Awareness during intubation performed with a muscle relaxant is distressing for the patient and can usually be overcome by pretreatment with a benzodiazepine such as Diazemuls or midazolam.

The effects of succinyl choline wear off in about 5 minutes. If the tube is not well tolerated and spontaneous ventilation is unsatisfactory then ventilation will have to be controlled using a longer acting non-depolarizing relaxant, for example vecuronium with opiate analgesia if appropriate.

In patients with a jeopardized airway due to maxillofacial injury it can be very dangerous to use muscle relaxants as airway control may be completely lost and the resulting apnoea may not be able to be replaced by artificial ventilation. On the other hand, the muscle relaxant may make intubation easier. Each case requires the individual expert clinical judgment of an experienced anaesthetist.

Opiates should not be given to patients with head injuries.

Technique
1. Establish a reliable i.v. route.
2. Prepare loaded syringes: one each of succinyl choline 100mg and Diazemuls 10mg; or one each of midazolam 5mg, atropine 1.0mg and vecuronium 10mg.
3. Preoxygenate if not in extremis.
4. Apply cricoid pressure.
5. Attempt laryngoscopy and intubation.
6. If intubation is unsuccessful due to struggling: reoxygenate; Diazemuls 10mg or midazolam 5mg, and suxamethonium 100mg; reattempt intubation.
7. Check: tracheal tube position, cuff seal, chest movements, pulse rate.
8. If pulse rate <60: atropine 1.0mg.▪▪▪▪▪▪

......**9** If the tube is not tolerated or the ensuing spontaneous ventilation is inadequate: vecuronium 10mg followed by opiate analgesia if appropriate.

10 If intubation is unsuccessful due to the larynx being obscured from view: clear the oropharynx by suction and reassess the possibility of intubation.

11 Either reattempt intubation with or without a muscle relaxant.

12 Or abandon the attempt and reassess the need for intubation.

Cricothyrotomy

If endotracheal intubation proves impossible in a patient with maxillofacial or laryngeal injury then cricothyrotomy should be used to establish a potent airway. Inexperienced laryngoscopists may have to resort to cricothyrotomy before an experienced anaesthetist would. The technique for cricothyrotomy is described on pp.31-33.

Protocol for airway management

A protocol for airway management is shown in Figure 3.2.

BREATHING

The patient's chest should be fully exposed to assess ventilation. In trauma victims, ventilation may commonly be impaired by:

• Pulmonary contusion ± fractured ribs.
• Tension pneumothorax.
• Open pneumothorax.
• Haemothorax and pulmonary collapse.
• Aspiration of foreign material.
• Hypoventilation due to head or spinal injury.

All patients should receive a high inspired concentration of oxygen (F_1O_2 = 0.85). Inadequate volume exchange should be supported by ventilation using a self-inflating bag or automatic resuscitatior.

Resuscitative measures should be instigated on clinical grounds alone and should not await radiological investigation.

Pulmonary contusion

Pulmonary contusion arises as a result of blunt chest trauma and it is usually (but not invariably) accompanied by rib fractures.

Diagnostic features may include:

• Dyspnoea and tachypnoea >20/min.
• Pain on inspiration.
• Reduced chest movement on the affected side.
• Cyanosis in severe cases.
• Flail segment if ribs fractured in two places.

Treatment
• Oxygen therapy.
• Controlled ventilation if volume exchange is poor.
• Pain relief.
• Watch for pneumothorax.

Tension pneumothorax

A tension pneumothorax develops if a one-way valvular leak occurs into the pleural cavity. The leak is generally caused by a fractured rib penetrating the lung but may also arise from air entering the pleural cavity from outside through a chest-wall injury.

Tension pneumothorax is a life-threatening condition requiring immediate diagnosis and treatment.

A simple pneumothorax may be converted to a tension pneumothorax by positive pressure ventilation, particularly if PEEP is applied. Be on guard for this.

Diagnostic features may include:

• Dyspnoea and tachypnoea >20/min.
• Pain on inspiration.
• Reduced chest movement on the affected side.
• Reduced air entry on the affected side.
• Hyper-resonance with percussion on the affected side.
• Tracheal deviation away from the affected side.
• Cyanosis.
• Fall in cardiac output due to mediastinal displacement causing reduced venous return, sometimes with distended neck veins, and hypotension.

Treatment
The treatment of a suspected tension pneumothorax is oxygen therapy and immediate decompression of the pleural cavity by needle thoracostomy (Fig. 3.3).

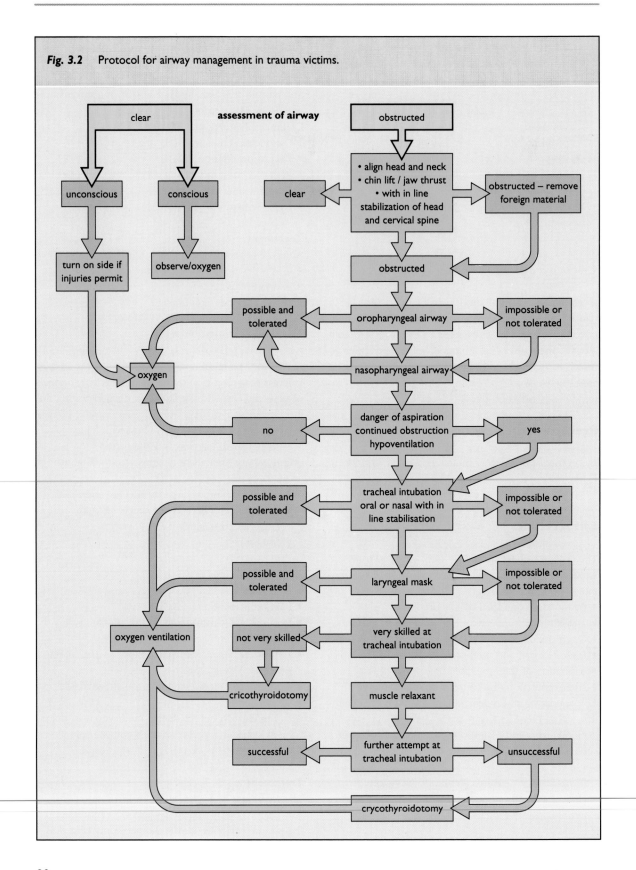

Fig. 3.2 Protocol for airway management in trauma victims.

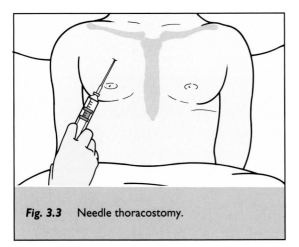

Fig. 3.3   Needle thoracostomy.

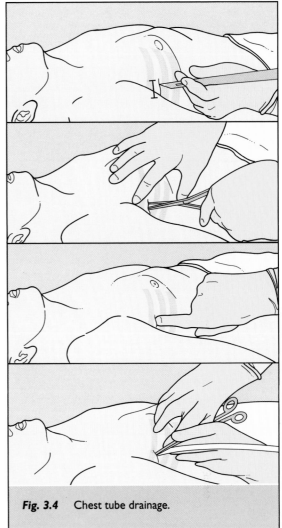

Fig. 3.4   Chest tube drainage.

Technique – needle thoracostomy

1 Insert a 16G i.v. cannula through the second intercostal space in the midclavicular line.

2 Listen for escaping air.

3 Remove the needle from inside the cannula, aspirate air with a syringe.

4 Leave the cannula *in situ* if air is aspirated.

5 If air is aspirated then chest tube drainage should be performed (Fig. 3.4).

Technique — chest tube drainage

1 Prepare the skin with antiseptic solution over the fifth intercostal space in the midaxillary line.

2 In conscious patients inject 2–5ml of lignocaine 2% into the proposed site subcutaneously down to the parietal pleura.

3 Make a 2cm incision in the skin over the upper border of the sixth rib (Fig. 3.4A).

4 Probe the incision with blunt forceps (Fig. 3.4B) seeking a path into the pleural cavity over the upper border of the sixth rib (note: the intercostal vessels and nerve lie beneath the lower border of the ribs).

5 Introduce a finger through the incision (Fig. 3.4C) into the pleural cavity and sweep around to ensure that the lung is not adherent to the chest wall. ●●●●●●

●●●●●**6** Grasping the chest tube (size 28–30FG) with the forceps, introduce it cephalad into the pleural cavity (Fig. 3.4D), ensuring that all side drainage holes are well within the cavity and not in, or outside, the chest wall.

7 Connect the chest tube to an underwater seal (Fig. 3.5) or to a chest drainage bag with built in flap valve (Fig. 3.6).

8 Secure the tube firmly to the skin with sutures placed at either end of the incision.

9 Support ventilation as required.

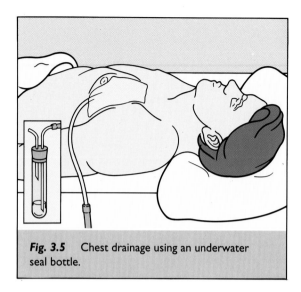

Fig. 3.5 Chest drainage using an underwater seal bottle.

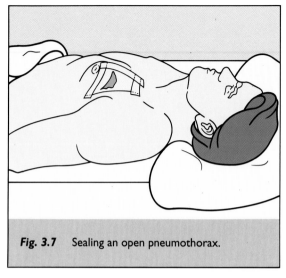

Fig. 3.7 Sealing an open pneumothorax.

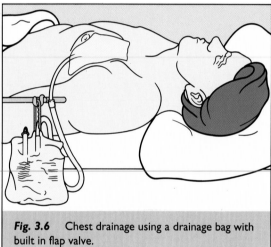

Fig. 3.6 Chest drainage using a drainage bag with built in flap valve.

Open pneumothorax

An open pneumothorax occurs as a result of an injury to the chest wall which penetrates into the pleural cavity.

Diagnostic features may include:
- An open wound of the chest wall.
- Dyspnoea and tachypnoea >20/min.
- Signs of pneumothorax — reduced chest movement and air entry and hyper-resonance on the affected side.
- Signs of haemothorax — reduced chest movement and air entry and dullness to percussion on the affected side.
- Signs of blood loss in severe cases.
- Cyanosis in severe cases.

Treatment
- Oxygen therapy.
- Cover the wound with an airtight dressing sealed on three sides to prevent air entering the pleural cavity but allowing the air inside under tension to escape into the atmosphere (Fig. 3.7).
- Insert a chest drain away from the injury site, preferably in the fifth intercostal space in the midaxillary line.
- Support ventilation as required.

Haemothorax

Haemothorax arises from penetrating or blunt chest trauma causing blood to accumulate in the pleural cavity with adjacent lung collapse.

Diagnostic features may include:
- Signs of blood loss (see pp.83–86).
- Dyspnoea and tachypnoea >20/min.
- Reduced chest movement and air entry and dullness to percussion on the affected side.
- Cyanosis in severe cases.

Treatment
- Oxygen therapy.
- Replace blood loss.
- Chest tube drainage through the fifth intercostal space in the midaxillary line, if lung collapse is more than 15 per cent.

• Consider exploratory thoracotomy if the blood loss initially is more than one litre or the continuing loss is greater than 200ml/h (thoracotomy is actually rarely required).

Aspiration of foreign material

This commonly occurs in trauma victims with an unprotected airway.
Diagnostic features may include:
• Dyspnoea and tachypnoea >20/min.
• Cyanosis in severe cases.
• Moist breath sounds and bronchospasm.

Treatment
• Oxygen therapy.
• Tracheal intubation.
• Tracheobronchial suction.
• Support ventilation as required.

Hypoventilation or apnoea

Hypoventilation may occur due to head or spinal injury. The treatment is positive pressure ventilation with added oxygen via an endotracheal tube.

Multiple lesions

It is important to remember that ventilation may be impaired by a number of factors; for instance haemo- and pneumothorax often occur together, and both may be compounded by pulmonary contusion or hypoventilation due to a severe head injury.

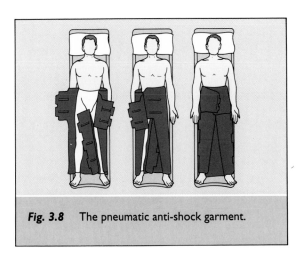

Fig. 3.8 The pneumatic anti-shock garment.

Chest radiology

Resuscitation requirements should be based on clinical grounds alone and not be dependent on positive findings from a chest X-ray. Unless radiology facilities are immediately available in the emergency room, a chest X-ray should be delayed until resuscitation has resulted in stable vital signs. The X-ray department that is distant from the emergency room is potentially a dangerous place.

CIRCULATION

Blood loss is the commonest remediable cause of morbidity and mortality after trauma. Successful management depends on the recognition of the presence and degree of hypovolaemia, the control of bleeding and the restoration of lost volume.
Early resuscitation should be based on the following observations:

■ STATE OF CONSCIOUSNESS:
Consciousness is impaired when 50 per cent or more of the circulating blood volume is lost.

■ SKIN COLOUR AND TEMPERATURE:
The skin is ashen grey centrally and white peripherally when 30 per cent or more of the circulating blood volume is lost.

■ THE PULSE:
The pulse becomes rapid and thready when 20 per cent or more of the circulating blood volume is lost. These signs indicate serious blood loss and immediate steps should be taken to control bleeding, replace lost volume and give oxygen therapy while a more detailed assessment of the degree of hypovolaemic shock is made.

Control of bleeding

Bleeding should be controlled by the first-aid measures of direct pressure on accessible wounds in the scalp, neck and limbs, and elevation of the bleeding part where possible. Tourniquets are not normally recommended. Blind clamping of bleeding points is hazardous. Serious haemorrhage in the limbs, pelvis and lower abdomen may be controlled by the application of a pneumatic anti-shock garment (PASG; medical anti-shock trousers, MAST) (Fig. 3.8).

Use of the pneumatic anti-shock garment

The effects of application are:

- An autotransfusion of 500–1000ml of autologous venous blood from the limbs and pelvis into the central circulation.
- Tamponade of bleeding vessels.
- An increase in peripheral vascular resistance in the arterial tree below pelvic level.
- Splintage of lower limb and pelvic fractures.
- The garment is radiotranslucent and has apertures for urinary catheterization and rectal and vaginal examination.

Technique

1 Apply the limb sections, first securing Velcro fittings together firmly.
2 Apply the abdominal section.
3 Inflate limb sections, followed by the abdominal section, to 80–100mmHg or until the Velcro fittings start to part.
4 Maintain volume replacement.
5 Observe the haemodynamic response.
6 Potential hazards and complications are associated with the application of the PASG.
7 Untimely removal will result in profound circulatory collapse. Once inflated the garment should not be deflated until the patient is in the operating room and volume replacement has been achieved. Deflation should be done in stages, the abdominal section first followed by the limb sections in controlled sequence.
8 Diaphragmatic splinting may occur as the abdominal contents are displaced cephalad and spontaneous ventilation may be impeded. The garment should not be used if diaphragmatic rupture is suspected.
9 Congestive cardiac failure may occur if the garment has been mistakenly applied to a patient with cardiogenic shock.
10 Increased intracranial pressure may develop in patients with normal blood volumes.
11 Crush injury, the compartment syndrome, and metabolic acidosis may occur if the garment is left inflated for too long. A limit of two hours should be adhered to.
12 The application of the garment should not delay intravenous volume replacement.

Assessment of lost volume

Volume replacement should be started immediately the simple signs of significant hypovolaemia have been detected. A minimum of two wide-bore (10–14G) i.v. lines should be established and transfusion commenced while a detailed assessment of the volume lost and rate of ongoing bleeding is made.

Pathophysiology

Compensatory haemodynamic changes occur in response to blood loss. Blood pressure is preserved initially by vasoconstriction in the splanchnic, cutaneous and muscle circulations. Hypotension occurs later as blood loss continues and cardiac output cannot be maintained. Tachycardia is the earliest sign of blood loss. At cellular level the reduced perfusion results in anaerobic metabolism and the development of metabolic acidosis.

The normal blood volume in adults is 7 per cent of body weight (5l/70kg). In children the blood volume proportion is slightly higher (8–9 per cent, or 80–90ml/kg).

Types of shock occurring after injury:

Four types of shock may be associated with injury:
- Hypovolaemic.
- Cardiogenic.
- Neurogenic.
- Septic.

Hypovolaemic shock

Hypovolaemic shock is the commonest type occurring after injury. The hypovolaemia is not only due to loss from the intravascular compartment but also due to oedema which accompanies soft tissue injury. Oedema fluid comes primarily from the interstitial compartment but, because the plasma is in equilibrium with the interstitial fluid, it may be estimated that 25 per cent of oedema fluid is contributed from the intravascular compartment. Hypovolaemic shock is revealed by the following diagnostic features:
- Skin: pallor, cool.
- Mental state: anxious, aggressive, confused, drowsy, unconscious.
- Circulation: tachycardia, reduced pulse pressure, reduced systolic and diastolic pressure, reduced central venous pressure.
- Respiration: tachypnoea.
- Urine flow: reduced.

The symptoms may be correlated with the degree of haemorrhage, but certain factors may modify the diagnostic features associated with a particular blood loss. These include:

- Patient age: signs more exaggerated with age.
- Injury severity: signs more exaggerated with extensive tissue damage.
- Previous medication: signs may be modified or masked (e.g. β–blockers prevent tachycardia, etc).
- Pre-hospital fluid replacement: may modify clinical signs.

As blood loss progresses, clinical signs and symptoms develop which can aid volume loss assessment. Degrees of haemorrhage (Fig. 3.9) may be allocated into four classes.

■ CLASS I HAEMORRHAGE — 15 PER CENT LOSE (750ml):
Losses up to 750ml do not produce any clinical signs or symptoms except for a slight tachycardia. The loss of blood volume is rapidly restored by compensatory fluid transfer and oral fluids.

■ CLASS II HAEMORRHAGE — 15–30 PER CENT (800–1500ml):
There is a tachycardia and a fall in pulse pressure due principally to a rise in diastolic pressure as a result of catecholamine release. The capillary refill test is prolonged (>2 seconds) and the patient may be anxious or aggressive. The urine flow rate is slightly reduced.

Such blood loss requires intravenous fluid replacement but blood transfusion will only be required in certain patients, (e.g. those with multiple injuries, pre-existing disease or haemoglobin reduction and the elderly).

■ CLASS III HAEMORRHAGE — 30–40 PER CENT (1500–2000ml):
It is at this stage that compensatory measures fail.

Fig. 3.9 Hypovolaemic shock: degrees of haemorrhage.

	class I	class II	class III	class IV
blood loss				
percentage	<15	15–30	30–40	>40
volume (ml)	750	800–1500	1500–2000	>2000
blood pressure				
systolic	unchanged	normal	reduced	very low
diastolic	unchanged	raised	reduced	very low or unrecordable
pulse	slight tachycardia	>100/min	120/min, thready	>120/min, very thready
capillary refill test	normal	slow (>2s)	slow (>2s)	undetectable
respiratory rate	normal	normal	tachypnoea (>20/min)	tachypnoea (>20/min)
urine flow rate (ml/hour)	>30	20–30	10–20	0–10
extremities	colour normal	pale	pale	pale and cold
complexion	normal	pale	pale	ashen
mental state	alert	anxious or aggressive	anxious, aggressive or drowsy	drowsy, confused, unconscious

There is a marked tachycardia, tachypnoea and a fall in both systolic and diastolic pressures. The patient is anxious, aggressive or drowsy with a pale complexion and extremities. Urinary output is considerably reduced.

This degree of loss requires immediate intravenous fluid replacement and subsequent blood transfusion.

■ **CLASS IV HAEMORRHAGE — >40 PER CENT (>2000ml):**
This degree of blood loss is life-threatening. There is a marked tachycardia, a profound fall in systolic and diastolic pressure (the latter may be unrecordable). The extremities are cold and pale and the complexion ashen, and the patient is confused and drowsy. Consciousness may be lost when the blood volume falls to 50 per cent. Urine output is scanty.

Such patients require rapid i.v. volume replacement, blood transfusion and, frequently, immediate surgery to control bleeding in the chest, abdomen or pelvis.

■ **THE CHANGING STATE IN INJURY**
The signs and symptoms, given above, for hypovolaemic shock are only a guideline to volume loss and transfusion requirements. Blood and fluid loss are likely to be continual during resuscitation, and the fluid replacement requirement must be determined by haemodynamic and other responses rather than being a predetermined estimate of the loss.

In addition to observations of the pulse, systolic and diastolic pressure, skin perfusion, mental state, etc., invaluable guides to the response to transfusion are the urine flow rate and central venous pressure (CVP). Adequate transfusion is indicated by:
- A urine flow rate of 50ml/h.
- A CVP which increases 2-3cmH$_2$O or more in response to a fluid challenge of 250–500ml.

Cardiogenic shock

Cardiogenic shock can occur after injury due to myocardial dysfunction arising as a result of cardiac contusion or tamponade, tension pneumothorax, air embolus, or myocardial infarction occurring at the time of injury in a patient with pre-existing myocardial ischaemia.

Myocardial contusion occurs as a result of blunt chest trauma. Cardiac tamponade is due to penetrating trauma. The signs and symptoms of cardiogenic shock are similar to those of hypovolaemic shock in that circulatory failure occurs. The principle differentiating signs between hypovolaemic shock and cardiogenic shock are:
- Central venous pressure: low in hypovolaemic shock, raised in cardiogenic shock.
- Skin colour: very pale in hypovolaemic shock, less pale in cardiogenic shock.
- ECG: injury pattern in myocardial contusion, no injury pattern in hypovolaemic shock.
- Isoenzymes: abnormal in myocardial contusion, normal in hypovolaemic shock.
- Ultrasound studies of the heart: abnormal in myocardial contusion, normal in hypovolaemic shock.
- Haematocrit: normal in cardiogenic shock, may be low in hypovolaemic shock.

Isoenzymes and ultrasound studies are not suitable for urgent diagnosis in the emergency situation. Haematocrit readings are unreliable as a reflection of acute blood loss.

Neurogenic shock
Neurogenic shock arises as a result of head injury. Isolated head injuries without severe scalp or maxillofacial wounds do not cause hypovolaemic shock.

In neurogenic shock, hypotension occurs but without tachycardia or vasoconstriction because of disruption of the sympathetic pathways descending in the cervical and upper thoracic spinal cord. As a result there is a loss of vasomotor tone, and there is no neural sympathetic stimulation of the heart. In contrast to severe hypovolaemia, the hypotension can be corrected by elevation of the legs and bradycardia relieved by atropine or a sympathomimetic agent (e.g. ephedrine or phenylephrine).

Despite the distinctions between different types of shock it should be remembered that in the clinical situation a given patient may exhibit more than one type, by suffering a combination of head injury, chest injury and abdominal or limb injuries. In these conditions the clinical signs require very careful evaluation.

Septic shock
Septic shock does not occur in the early stages after trauma. The management of this condition therefore is outside the scope of this handbook.

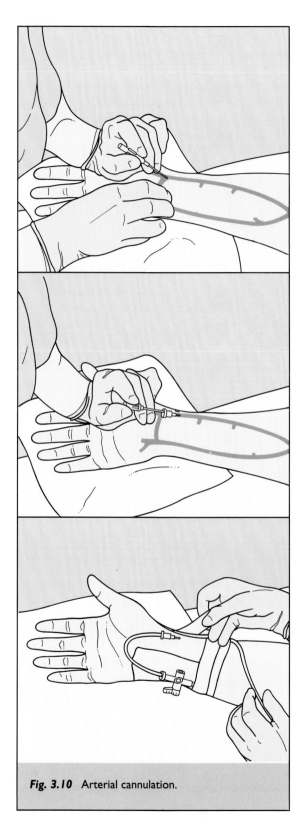

Fig. 3.10 Arterial cannulation.

Arterial blood pressure measurement

Arterial blood pressure is a key, vital sign in all patients with shock. Initially the pressure will be measured using a non-invasive sphygomanometer, but in all cases of severe shock and major injury an arterial cannula should be inserted to provide a continual read out of systolic, diastolic and mean pressures (Fig. 3.10).

Technique

1   Prepare the skin over the radial artery with an antiseptic solution.
2   Hyperextend the wrist by placing a one-litre bag of intravenous fluid beneath the dorsum of the wrist.
3   Palpate the radial artery.
4   Inject a "bleb" of 1% lignocaine into the skin over the artery.
5   Make a small skin incision with a scalpel blade.
6   Using a 20G cannula-over-needle, make an arterial puncture through the skin incision. Successful puncture is indicated by a free spontaneous flow of blood into the cannula hub.
7   Twist and rotate the cannula over the needle up into the arterial lumen.
8   Compress the artery proximal to the cannula tip, and attach the cannula hub via a three-way tap to the primed manometer line leading to the pressure transducer.
9   Release the arterial compression and check for the arterial trace on the oscilloscope.
10 Secure the cannula tap and manometer line with an adhesive dressing and tape.

Replacement of colume loss: Venous access

Venous access may be gained by a peripheral or central route; the choice of which to use is dictated by a number of factors:
- Availability of accessible vein.
- Site of injury.
- Training and competence of the operator.
- Availability of the appropriate equipment.

The peripheral route

The peripheral route is the simplest to establish and requires only the most basic of equipment. The veins of the arm are accessible in most cases, and cannulation there carries less risk of venous thrombosis than cannulae placed in the veins of the leg. Patients with abdominal trauma may have injury to veins in the pelvis or abdomen, and infused fluids from the leg veins may leak extravascularily.

In most patients there is a choice of veins in the arm (Fig. 3.11). The best sites to choose are the radial aspect of the wrist, the dorsum of the hand or the cephalic vein in the upper arm, as they are not directly situated over joints and the cannula is less likely to be displaced. The more peripheral sites should be selected first so that a more proximal site is still available in case of failure or displacement.

In some patients the veins of the antecubital fossa will be the only accessible ones. If this site is used the arm should be splinted to avoid cannula displacement by elbow flexion.

In all cases of major trauma at least two sites should be cannulated.

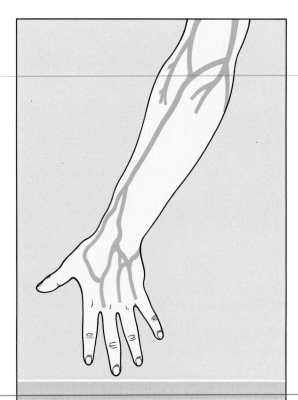

Fig. 3.11 Venous access sites in the arm.

■ **SELECTION OF CANNULA**

Flow rates through cannulae are inversely related to the length of the cannula and directly related to the fourth power of the radius (r^4). Therefore intravenous cannulae should be short and of as wide a diameter as can be inserted into the vein. The "cannula-over-needle" is the best type to select. A 14G cannula is the minimum diameter necessary for rapid transfusion of packed red cells or whole blood. A 16G cannula will be adequate for blood substitutes. Cannulae with a built-in port allow for easy injection of drugs — otherwise a three-way tap must be interposed between the cannula and giving set (Fig. 3.12). The resealable site in the giving set is unsuitable as it may leak after being punctured if the infusion is given under pressure.

Technique for peripheral intravenous cannulation

1   Identify the vein to be cannulated by circumferential compression of the limb proximal to the site, either by an assistant using their hands or by using a tourniquet. The pressure used should not exceed arterial pressure.
2   A site where there is a 'Y' pattern of veins (see Fig. 3.11) is the most suitable as skin puncture can be made away from the vein.
3   Prepare the skin over the selected site with an antiseptic solution.
4   Pierce the skin and insert the needle into the vein for 1cm so that the cannula part lies securely within the vein lumen (Fig. 3.13A). Insertion into the vein will be indicated by a "flash back" of blood into the cannula hub.
5   Withdraw the needle back into the cannula for 1cm (Fig. 3.13B).
6   Holding the needle steady push the cannula up the vein until the hub reaches the skin.
7   Compress the vein above the end of the cannula (Fig. 3.13C).
8   Remove the needle and attach the giving set which has been primed and flushed to remove air.
9   Release venous compression and check the flow through the giving set.
10 Ensure that no extravasation has occurred at the venepuncture site.
11 Secure the cannula and giving set with adhesive dressing and tape (Fig. 3.13D).

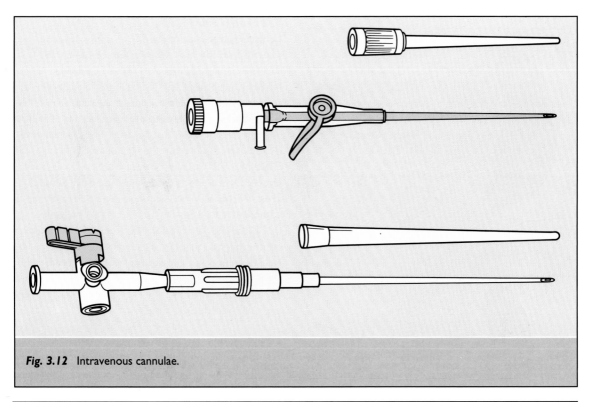

Fig. 3.12 Intravenous cannulae.

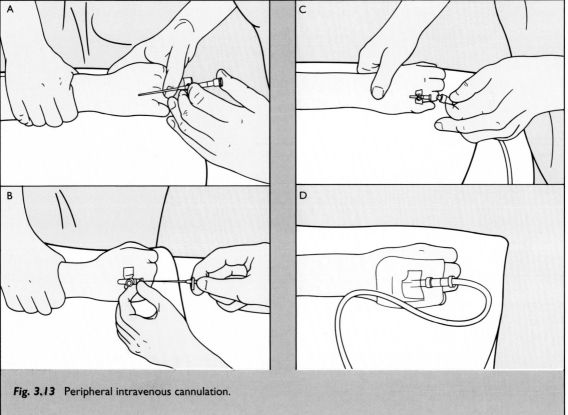

Fig. 3.13 Peripheral intravenous cannulation.

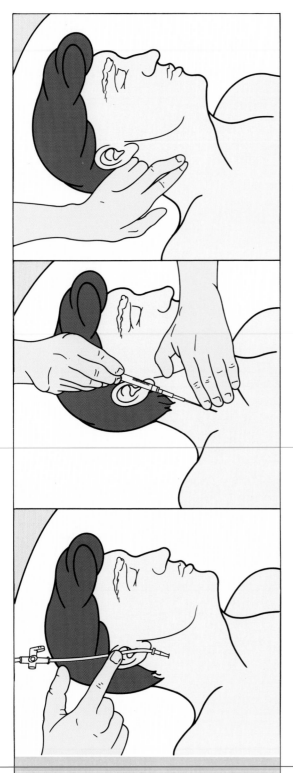

Fig. 3.14 Cannulation of the internal jugular vein.

The central route

Central venous cannulation requires training and expertise on the part of the operator but carries with it considerable advantages in many instances. Larger bore 10G cannulae can be inserted and more than one cannula can be placed into the same vein. The route from central veins to the heart is short and fluid or drug therapy has a rapid effect. Once the expertise is acquired the technique is reliable because the anatomical disposition of the central veins is consistent (except in the case of the external jugular). A centrally placed venous cannula may be connected to a transducer to measure central venous pressure.

The commonly chosen sites for central cannulation are the internal jugular or the subclavian veins or by long line through the antecubital fossa and, occasionally, the femoral vein. The choice depends largely on the operator's preference, the site of injury and area of proposed surgery.

■ **CANNULATION OF THE INTERNAL JUGULAR VEIN**
The internal jugular vein may be cannulated in the neck as it lies beneath the confluence of the sternal and clavicular heads of the sternocleidomastoid muscle (Fig. 3.14). The vein on the right side is commonly chosen for preference.

Technique
1 Place the patient supine, head-down at 15°, and turn the head to the left.

Do not rotate the head in patients with suspected cervical spine injuries.

2 Prepare the skin with an antiseptic solution.
3 Identify the confluence of the two heads of the sternocleidomastoid muscle.
4 Palpate the common carotid artery.
5 Using a 7.5–12.5cm long cannula-over-needle of 10–14G diameter with a 5ml syringe attached, pierce the skin just lateral to the carotid artery at an angle of 30°, directing the cannula towards the ipsilateral nipple.
6 Venepuncture is confirmed by free flow aspiration of blood into the syringe and should occur once the needle has advanced up to 3–4cm from the skin surface, depending on the patient's corpulence. ■■■■■■

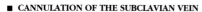7 Lower the syringe to make a more acute angle with the skin and twist and advance the cannula over the needle and into the vein until the hub reaches the skin.

8 Withdraw the needle and check free aspiration of blood through the cannula.

9 Connect the primed giving set to the cannula via a three-way tap.

10 Secure the cannula, tap and giving set, with an adhesive dressing and tape.

11 A second or third cannula can be inserted into the same vein for extra transfusion potential or for connection to a central venous pressure monitor.

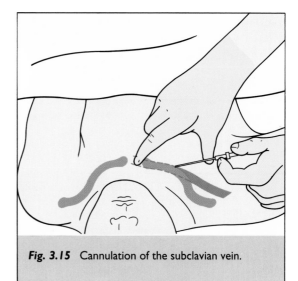

Fig. 3.15 Cannulation of the subclavian vein.

■ CANNULATION OF THE SUBCLAVIAN VEIN

The subclavian vein may be cannulated as it emerges from the thorax over the first rib and beneath the clavicle (Fig. 3.14).

Technique

1 Place the patient supine with a 15° head-down tilt.

2 Prepare the skin with an antiseptic solution.

3 Identify the clavicle and suprasternal notch by palpation.

4 Using a 7.5–12.5cm cannula-over-needle of 10–14G diameter with a 5ml syringe attached, pierce the skin 1cm below the junction of the medial and middle thirds of the clavicle (Fig. 3.15).

5 Advance the cannula and needle just beneath the clavicle and over the first rib, aiming towards the opposite shoulder at a finger placed in the suprasternal notch.

6 Venepuncture is confirmed by free flow aspiration of blood into the syringe and should occur once the needle has advanced 3–4cm from the skin surface.

7 Twist and advance the cannula over the needle until the hub reaches the skin.

8 Withdraw the needle and check free aspiration of blood through the cannula.

9 Connect the primed giving set to the cannula via a three-way tap.

10 Secure the cannula, tap and giving set with an adhesive dressing and tape.

11 Check the cannula position by X-ray.

The apical pleura lies close to the subclavian vein as it crosses the first rib. Accidental pneumothorax is a distinct possibility due to needle puncture of the pleura and should be looked for on the X-ray check.

■ CANNULATION OF THE INTERNAL JUGULAR OR SUBCLAVIAN VEINS USING THE SELDINGER TECHNIQUE

Cannulation of the internal or the subclavian veins may also be performed using the Seldinger principle (Fig. 3.16). Single, multilumen or pulmonary artery (Swan Ganz) catheters may be introduced using this technique.

Technique

1 Ensure cannulation kit is complete and prepared.

2 Place the patient supine, prepare the skin and identify landmarks as before.

3 Make venepuncture with needle attached to a 5ml syringe.

4 Remove syringe and pass guide wire down needle.

5 Remove needle.

6 Make a 0.25cm incision in skin (and platysma for jugular vein). ■■■■■

7 Pass dilator(s) over guide wire into vein.

8 Pass catheter into vein over guide wire.

9 Remove guide wire.

10 Secure in position and attach to giving set and/or manometer tubing.

11 Check catheter position on X-ray.

■ **CENTRAL VENOUS CANNULATION VIA BRACHIAL VEIN IN THE ANTECUBITAL FOSSA**

This technique can be used by those unfamiliar with the internal jugular or subclavian route. A long catheter (70cm) over-needle is required and this length limits the flow rate. The cephalic vein in the antecubital fossa may also be used but is less

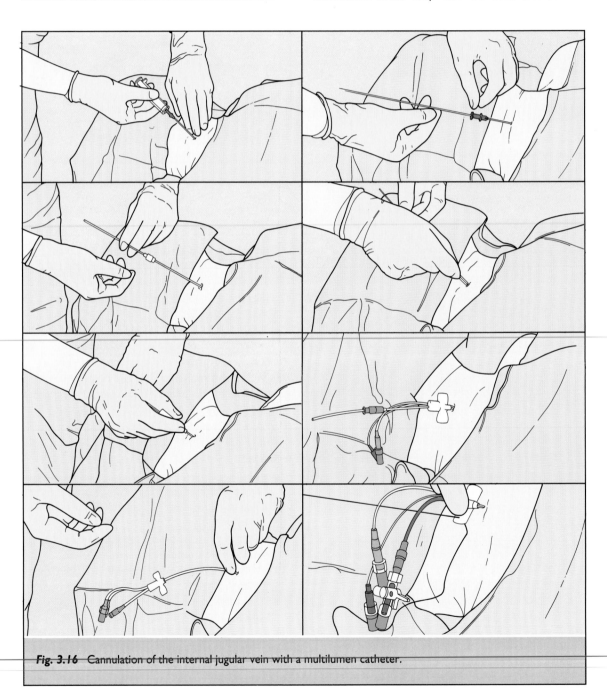

Fig. 3.16 Cannulation of the internal jugular vein with a multilumen catheter.

preferable because introduction of the catheter may be held up at the clavipectoral fascia.

Technique

1 Prepare the skin around the antecubital fossa with an antiseptic solution.
2 Palpate the brachial artery to identify its position and to ensure that it is not punctured inadvertently.
3 Identify the adjacent brachial vein by circumferential pressure applied around the upper arm.
4 Insert a 12–14G diameter cannula-over-needle into the vein as for peripheral venepuncture.
5 Remove the needle and advance the cannula fully into the vein.
6 Thread the catheter through the cannula into the vein and advance it until the tip is judged to have reached the superior vena cava.
7 Confirm that the catheter is in the venous system by aspirating a free flow of blood.
8 Connect the primed giving set to the catheter, check for infusion flow.
9 Secure the catheter and giving set with adhesive dressing and tape.
10 Check the catheter position in the superior vena cava on an X-ray.

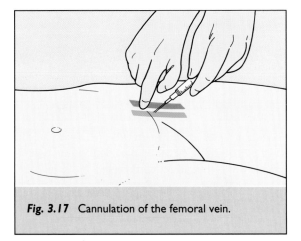

Fig. 3.17 Cannulation of the femoral vein.

■ CANNULATION OF THE FEMORAL VEIN

This route is preferred by some who consider it a more simple technique (Fig. 3.17). The femoral vein is also suitable for use with injuries around the pectoral girdle. However, it is more likely to become infected, and thrombo-embolism is more common from the pelvic and leg veins than from the jugular or subclavian system. Therefore cannulae or catheters placed in the femoral vein should not be left there for long periods of time. The route should not be used in patients with pelvic or abdominal injuries.

Technique

1 Palpate the femoral artery in the groin just below the inguinal ligament. The vein lies immediately medial to the artery.
2 Prepare the skin with an antiseptic solution.
3 Using a 7.5–12.5cm long cannula-over-needle of 10–14G diameter with a 5ml syringe attached pierce the skin 1cm medial to the femoral artery 2cm below the lower border of the inguinal ligament (Fig. 3.17).
4 Advance the needle and cannula cephalad at an angle of 30° until a free flow aspiration of blood occurs at 3-4cm.
5 Twist and advance the cannula over the needle. Withdraw the needle.
6 Confirm that the cannula lies within the vein by aspiration of blood.
7 Connect the primed giving set, incorporating a three-way tap, and check for free infusion flow.
8 Secure the cannula and giving set with adhesive dressing and taper.

■ VENOUS CUTDOWN

Occasionally, direct percutaneous peripheral or central venepuncture may prove impossible because of unavailable sites or lack of appropriate operator skill. In such cases venous access can be secured using a surgical cutdown method. The long saphenous vein at the ankle is generally used or alternatively the brachial vein in the antecubital fossa (Fig. 3.18).

In severe haemorrhage the long saphenous vein in the groin may be used and a wide bore nasogastric tube or the end of an infusion giving set (with the resealable port cut off) introduced directly for very rapid volume replacement.

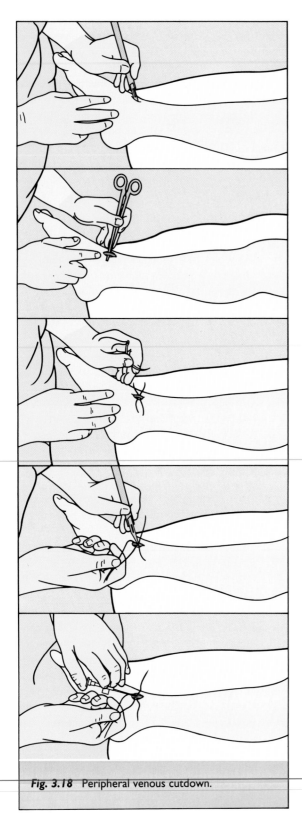

Fig. 3.18 Peripheral venous cutdown.

Technique

1 Identify the vein by circumferential compression of limb proximal to site.
2 Prepare the skin with an antiseptic solution.
3 Drape the site.
4 Make an incision in the skin over the vein (a longitudinal or transverse incision may be used as preferred; the longitudinal incision generally heals better).
5 Probe the incision with blunt forceps to identify the vein and free it from the subcutaneous tissues.
6 Pass a suture beneath the vein using an aneurysm needle or forceps.
7 Divide the suture to form loops proximally and distally around the proposed venepuncture site.
8 Maintaining tension over the distal loop, make a 2mm incision in the vein.
9 Probe this incision with the tip of fine-artery forceps to confirm access inside the vein lumen.
10 Insert the venous cannula (10–14G).
11 Tie the proximal loop over the cannula.
12 Attach the primed giving set and confirm free flow.
13 Remove the distal suture loop.
14 Suture the skin incision.
15 Secure the cannula hub and giving set with an adhesive dressing or tape.

Replacement of lost volume: Fluid therapy

Volume loss in hypovolaemia resulting from trauma can be replaced using crystalloids, colloids, packed red cells or whole blood.

In the majority of patients fluid replacement will be started using blood substitutes — either crystalloids or colloids or a mixture of both. In some patients with modest losses these substitutes alone will suffice. In patients with a loss of 25 per cent of their blood volume or more (≥1500ml), subsequent blood transfusion will generally be necessary. In calculating blood loss account must be taken of continuing losses — not just current losses.

Choice of blood substitute

There has been a continuing debate as to the relative merits of crystalloid or colloid as the best blood substitute in hypovolaemia. The proponents of crystalloid therapy argue that intravascular loss is also reflected by a depletion of extracellular fluid and that crystalloid will permeate into both of these compartments. Colloid supporters argue that these substances are retained in the intravascular compartment, maintain colloid osmotic pressure and improve haemodynamics more rapidly.

It is likely that a mixture of colloid and crystalloid provides optimal treatment. In severe blood loss (>30 per cent blood volume) fluid replacement should be started with colloid (1.0–1.5l), followed by a litre of crystalloid and then by equal amounts of colloid and crystalloid until blood is available.

■ AVAILABLE CRYSTALLOIDS

■ COMPOUND RINGER LACTATE SOLUTION (HARTMANN'S SOLUTION):

This solution is the most commonly used crystalloid. It is electrolytically isotonic with plasma and permeates readily into the extracellular spaces. The half-life of Hartmann's solution is short and it is rapidly excreted in the urine. If resuscitation with this solution alone is planned, a volume of 3–4 times the blood loss is required to restore normal haemodynamics.

■ HYPERTONIC SALINE SOLUTIONS:

6.0–7.5 per cent saline solutions have been used successfully to treat hypovolaemia particularly in burned patients. The hypertonic solution draws fluid from the extracellular space to enhance the intravascular volume and restore haemodynamics. A small volume therefore will have a relatively profound effect and, as such, has potential value in the pre-hospital phase where rapid restoration of the circulation is required. The dose of hypertonic saline should be limited to 500–750ml. The infusion can be given by the central or peripheral venous route.

■ AVAILABLE COLLOIDS

The action of intravenous colloids depends on their molecular weight and half-life duration. Substances with high molecular weight exert a high colloid osmotic pressure which restores haemodynamics but which may deplete the extracellular space. A long half-life ensures a long duration of action but this may create problems when intravascular "space" is required for blood transfusion later.

■ THE POLYGELATINS (HAEMACCEL AND GELOFUSINE):

These are the most commonly used colloid solutions in the UK and Europe. They are approximately electrolytically isotonic with plasma, although Gelofusine has less potassium and calcium. Both have the same pH as plasma, a half-life of 8–10 hours, a low incidence of anaphylactic reactions, a long shelf-life and are relatively inexpensive. They do not interfere with coagulation or blood group estimation.

■ THE DEXTRANS:

Dextrans are available in a range of molecular weights (mol.wt). Dextran 70 in 5 per cent dextrose (mol.wt 70,000) is the most commonly used product for hypovolaemia. It has a low pH (4.5), a half-life of about 16 hours, a fairly low but significant incidence of anaphylactic reactions and is also relatively inexpensive. Dextran 70 mixed with blood may cause rouleaux formation and complicate blood group estimation. Blood samples should therefore be taken prior to dextran infusion.

There is some uncertainty as to whether a proportion of Dextran 70 is retained in the reticular endothelial system and therefore most authorities prefer to restrict the volume infused to 1.0–1.5 litres.

Dextran 40 (mol.wt. 40,000) is rarely used for the treatment of hypovolaemia. Its principle recommended action is to improve the microcirculation through its action of causing red blood corpuscles to repel each other. In the injured patient however such an action might well cause an increase in bleeding.

■ HYDROXYETHYL STARCH (HETASTARCH, HESPAN):

The commonly used preparations of hydroxyethyl starch have a molecular weight of 120,000. The half-life is long (16–24 hours) and the product is therefore useful in moderate blood loss when blood availability is likely to be delayed. Conversely, however, transfusion with hydroxyethyl starch may produce a replenished intravascular volume but a low haematocrit. Blood transfusion aimed at correcting the low haematocrit may then cause circulatory overload reflected by a markedly increased central venous pressure.

Hydroxyethyl starch has a low incidence of anaphylactic reaction, does not interfere with blood grouping and has a long shelf-life, but it is considerably more expensive than the polygelatin solutions.

■ HUMAN ALBUMEN SOLUTION:

Human albumen solution potentially is the ideal plasma substitute exerting a physiologically colloid osmotic pressure. However it has a number of drawbacks — it is expensive and carries a very small risk of anaphylaxis and infection. In most cases therefore it has little advantage over the polygelatins. Like other colloid solutions it does not replenish losses from the extracellular space and therefore should be used in conjunction with crystalloid.

■ OXYGEN-CARRYING BLOOD SUBSTITUTES:

The ideal blood substitute should be capable of carrying oxygen in a manner similar to haemoglobin. The search for such a product continues.

The perfluorocarbons (e.g. Fluosol DA) do in fact carry oxygen, but in a linear fashion, unlike haemoglobin which is designed for physiological oxygen uptake and release (Fig. 3.19). Thus exposure to a very high F_1O_2 is required for any useful oxygen carrying capacity. This limits its practical value. The product must be stored in a deep-frozen state. There is some doubt about whether a proportion is retained in the body and most authorities therefore limit infusions to one litre. Fluosol cannot be recommended for widespread clinical use, although it is possible that another perfluorocarbon molecule may be developed which could be more suitable.

Stroma-free haemoglobin and frozen blood are potential oxygen carrying materials but considerable further research and refinement is required before they can be introduced into clinical practice.

Blood

Blood is available as either whole blood or packed red cells. Blood transfusion is essential where losses exceed two litres. Fresh blood (1-day-old) retains red cell and platelet integrity to a large degree, but these elements disintegrate over a period of four weeks. Platelets in particular have a very short shelf-life.

While blood is essential in all cases of substantial loss it does carry some drawbacks. Tissue perfusion is better with a reduced haemotocrit (30 per cent), and therefore modest losses of up to one litre are best treated with a colloid/crystalloid mixture. Although the risk is small, there remains a chance of mismatch, infection and reaction with every blood transfusion. Blood is very expensive in comparison with artificial colloid solutions.

Practical aspects of transfusion

■ TEMPERATURE AND TRANSFUSION RATES

The rapid infusion of cold fluids may cause arrhythmias and core hypothermia. Such problems are particularly associated with blood which is stored at 4°C. Blood therefore should be warmed to 37°C prior to transfusion. Other fluids should be warmed if given rapidly and in all hypothermic patients.

The Level One transfusion device (Fig. 3.20) is designed to warm i.v. fluids speedily and effectively. Very rapid transfusion rates (one litre in four minutes) can be achieved provided wide bore venous access is available. At least two 10–14G cannulae should be used with pressure infusors to provide high flow rates.

■ FILTRATION

The use of filters to remove "debris" from stored blood has been advocated by some but clinical trials have failed to show any real positive benefit.

■ GIVING SETS

The same giving set should not be used for blood and other colloids such as the polygelatins and hydroxyethyl starch.

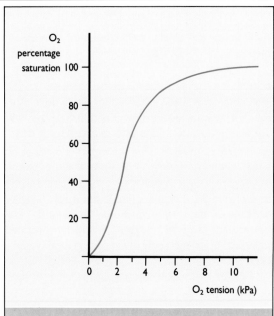

Fig. 3.19 The Bohr dissociation curve.

■ **CIRCULATORY OVERLOAD**

Circulatory overload can occur if excessive volumes are transfused. The situation is most likely to develop in patients with incipient or frank cardiac failure. The signs of circulatory overload are the development of pulmonary oedema and a rising central venous pressure in response to a low volume fluid challenge. All patients having substantial transfusions should be monitored with a central venous pressure line. The simultaneous measurement of pulmonary artery wedge pressure through a pulmonary artery flotation catheter can help in differentiating between left and right ventricular failure, but it is rarely of practical use in the early stages of resuscitation of the injured.

Circulatory overload should be treated by diuretics (e.g. frusemide 40–120mg), inotropes (e.g. dopamine $5\mu g/kg/h$) and intermittent positive pressure ventilation with PEEP (in severe cases of pulmonary oedema). Successful treatment is rewarded by a substantial increase in the urine flow rate.

■ **COAGULATION PROBLEMS**

Coagulation problems are rare during the first hour of resuscitation of the injured. If massive transfusion is contemplated it is good practice to take baseline measurements of prothrombin time, partial thromboplastin time and platelet count early on to assess any pre-existing coagulation defects.

Coagulation problems occurring after transfusion of large volumes should be analyzed carefully in conjunction with the haematology department. Blind use of platelets and fresh frozen plasma is costly and may not achieve the desired effect in dilutional coagulopathy.

Surgical intervention

Although it is desirable to correct hypovolaemia prior to surgery, this is not always possible in patients with substantial ongoing haemorrhage into the chest, abdomen or pelvis. In such patients the decision should be made to embark immediately on surgical control of the bleeding. Experienced anaesthetists and surgeons are required and intervention must be rapid. Once bleeding is controlled, definitive surgical repair of the damaged tissues should be delayed while the circulating blood volume and haemodynamics are restored by transfusion.

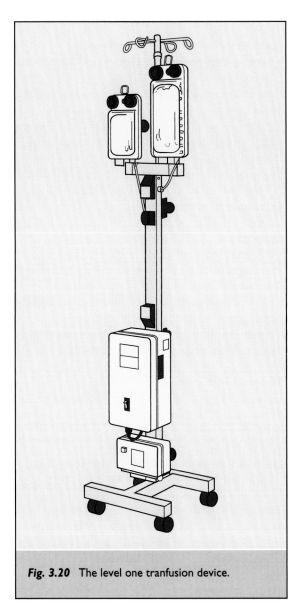

Fig. 3.20 The level one tranfusion device.

THE SECONDARY SURVEY

Once the primary survey has been completed, the cervical spine has been stabilized and life-threatening problems in the airway, breathing and the circulation have been corrected, the patient should be briefly assessed neurologically and then undressed for a thorough clinical examination — the secondary survey. This survey should proceed in an orderly sequence to ensure that no injury is missed.

NEUROLOGICAL ASSESSMENT

A brief neurological assessment should be carried out in all patients before the full secondary survey is started.

The object of this assessment is purely to ascertain the patient's level of consciousness and pupil size. A deteriorating level of consciousness may be due to hypoxia, hypercarbia or hypovolaemia, as well as head injury. The AVPU system advocated by the American College of Surgeons in its *Advanced Trauma Life Support Course Manual* is appropriate for this rapid assessment of conscious level:

> A – Alert.
> V – Responds to vocal stimuli.
> P – Responds to painful stimuli.
> U – Unresponsive.

The pupils are assessed for size, equality and reaction to light.

As the Secondary Survey proceeds a full neurological examination is carried out along the lines of the Glasgow Coma Scale (GCS) (see pp.98–99).

The head

Cervical spine injury should be suspected in all patients with a serious head injury.

The head should be carefully examined for:
- Palpable depressed skull fractures and scalp lacerations.
- Signs of cerebrospinal fluid (CSF) leakage from the ears or nose.
- Evidence of eye injury — conjunctiva, cornea, pupil inequality, lens dislocation, fundal injury, visual defect.

All patients who have sustained a head injury should be continually reassessed in terms of their vital signs and neurological function.

Vital signs
- Hypertension, bradycardia and a fall in respiratory rate indicate a severe injury with rising intracranial pressure.
- Hypertension alone or with hyperthermia indicates brain injury causing autonomic dysfunction.
- Intracranial bleeding does not cause hypovolaemic shock. There is another source of bleeding.

Glasgow coma scale
A patient's GCS score is obtained by scanning the scores for eye opening, best motor response and verbal response (Fig. 3.21).

> Note: the verbal response score cannot be assessed if speech is impossible, (e.g. if the patient is intubated).

All patients with a GCS <8 are in coma and those with a GCS >8 are not in coma.
- GCS>8 indicates a severe head injury.
- GCS 9–12 indicates a moderate head injury.
- GCS 13–15 indicates a minor head injury.

Changes in GCS are particularly relevant in the patient assessment.

■ LATERALIZING LIMB WEAKNESS:
Lateralizing limb weakness may indicate an intracranial injury such as an extradural haematoma on the opposite side.

■ PUPIL FUNCTION:

Pupil function should be continually reassessed for size, equality and reaction to light. The pupils may both be dilated in the very early stages of concussion. A unilateral, fixed, dilated pupil usually indicates an intracranial lesion on the same side. Bilateral fixed dilated pupils indicate a most serious head injury. It should be remembered that pupil size may be affected by drugs, (e.g. (atropine, opiates, etc).

If the clinical examination indicates any head injury other than a trivial one, (e.g. GCS >13 with no lateralizing weakness, pupil abnormality, or signs of skull fracture), then a computerized tomography (CT) scan should be carried out to enable the injury to be localized and assessed for treatment by surgery, in the intensive care unit (ICU) or in the general ward.

Skull X-rays are of limited value in assisting with head injury management and their role has been largely taken over by CT scanning.

A summary of head injury assessment is given in Figure 3.22.

eye opening	score
spontaneous (normal)	4
to command	3
to pain	2
none	1
best motor response	
moves limbs to command normally	6
localizes painful stimulus	5
withdraws from painful stimulus	4
flexes with painful stimulus	3
extends with painful stimulus	2
no response to pain	1
verbal response	
orientated — name, age, etc.	5
confused answers to questions	4
inappropriate speech	3
incomprehensible grunts	2
no response	1

Fig. 3.21 The Glasgow Coma Scale.

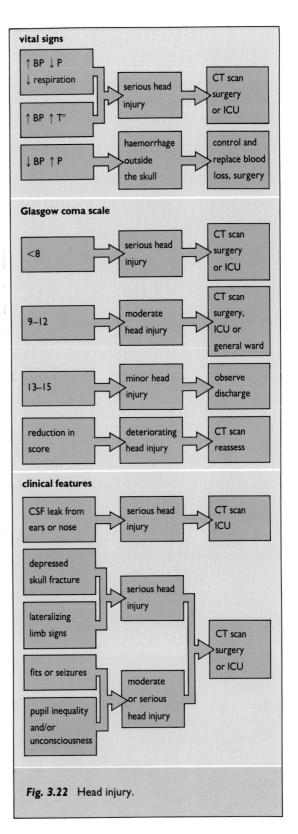

Fig. 3.22 Head injury.

The maxillofacial region

Maxillofacial injury without airway impairment or torrential haemorrhage is not life-threatening. Detailed assessment can wait until other injuries have been sought and the patient has been stabilized. Nevertheless an early evaluation of the injuries is important if the patient is to be treated for other injuries, particularly if anaesthesia and surgery is contemplated, because attempts at endotracheal intubation may cause sudden haemorrhage and loose teeth may be broken off and be inhaled or ingested.

It is also important to note any possible fracture of the cribriform plate because gastric intubation through the nose would be contraindicated, in case the tube might pass through the fracture site into the cranial cavity.

Cervical spine injury should be suspected in all patients with serious maxillofacial trauma.

The spine and neck

Cervical spine injury should be suspected in all patients suffering from serious blunt trauma above clavicular level.

The head, neck and shoulders should be stabilized in a neutral position by an assistant, while the airway is secured if necessary, and while an examination (Fig. 3.23) of the neck is made. Flexion and rotation are particularly dangerous movements. The neck should be stabilized using a spinal board, cervical collar and head, shoulder, hip and leg straps with padding wedges (Fig. 3.24) or a Hines splint (Fig. 3.25).

The absence of any relevant symptoms does not exclude cervical spine injury. The presence or absence of injury can only be confirmed by an X-ray showing all seven cervical vertebrae, using a "swimmers" or "shoot through" view if necessary. Neck immobilization should be maintained until injury is excluded by radiology and the absence of positive clinical signs.

X-ray films should be examined for:
- Anteroposterior diameter of the spinal canal.
- Contour and alignment of the vertebral bodies.
- Bone fragments – especially in the spinal canal.
- Fractures of the laminae, pedicles or neural arches.
- Soft tissue swelling.

Blunt trauma to the front of the neck may cause laryngeal or tracheal damage or haematoma formation which may result in airway obstruction. Penetrating trauma may cause severe haemorrhage, nerve damage or laryngeal, tracheal or oesophageal perforation.

The control of the airway, breathing and haemorrhage are of paramount importance and should be managed along the usual resuscitative lines. Increasing haematoma formation in the neck, impairing the airway, requires immediate surgical decompression.

Spinal injury below the cervical region

Spinal injury in the thoracolumbar region will be suspected in certain types of injury and in the light of the clinical signs detected. Thoracolumbar vertebral injuries commonly occur with falls from a height and in aircraft and road traffic accidents and should be suspected in all such incidents.

Conscious patients will generally be able to identify the site of injury because it is painful. Palpation of the spine will reveal tenderness and sometimes

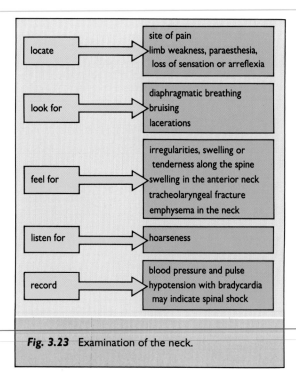

Fig. 3.23 Examination of the neck.

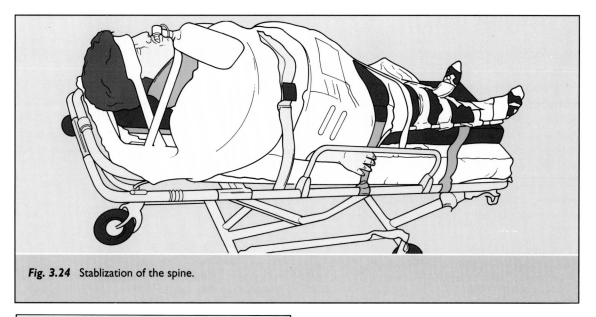

Fig. 3.24 Stablization of the spine.

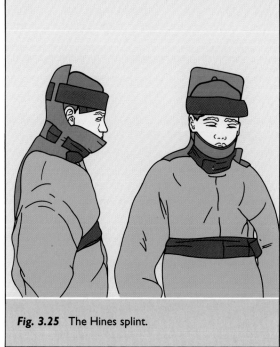

Fig. 3.25 The Hines splint.

swelling and deformity. In patients with spinal cord injury neurological symptoms occur below the injury level. A full neurological examination should be carried out looking for lower limb weakness, hyperaesthesia, loss of sensation and reflexes, priapism, and loss of rectal sphincter and bladder tone.

Neurogenic (spinal) shock (hypotension with a bradycardia) may be present due to impairment of the sympathetic pathways in the thoracolumbar region.

All patients with suspected spinal injuries should be immobilized from head to lower limbs pending confirmation by X-ray examination.

Anteroposterior and thoracic views of the thoracolumbar spine and sacrum should be taken amplified, if necessary, by CT scan or magnetic resonance imaging (MRI).

THE CHEST

The early assessment and management of the pulmonary consequences of chest trauma have been described on pp.79–83. The majority of pulmonary injuries can be treated conservatively with chest drainage, oxygenation and ventilatory support. Only five per cent require surgical intervention for continuing serious haemorrhage or major lung leak. Certain other consequences of chest injury however require consideration.

Penetrating cardiac injury

Penetrating injuries to the heart may result in cardiac tamponade. The diagnostic features of tamponade are:
- A penetrating wound.
- Hypotension.
- Tachycardia.
- Distended neck veins and a raised central venous pressure (CVP).
- Muffled heart sounds.

The condition is life-threatening and may be temporarily relieved by needle aspiration of the pericardium (Fig. 3.26). A tension pneumothorax may also be present.

> **Technique of needle pericardiocentesis**
> 1 Monitor arterial and CVP and the ECG.
> 2 Prepare xiphoid region with an antiseptic solution.
> 3 Instil lignocaine 1% into the skin puncture site 1cm below and just to the left of the xiphoid process.
> 4 Using a 16G cannula-over-needle with 20ml syringe and three-way tap attached, pierce the skin at a 30° angle aiming for the tip of the left shoulder.
> 5 Advance the needle while aspirating continually with the syringe until blood appears.
> 6 When blood appears remove the needle and attach the tap and syringe to the cannula. ■■■■■■

> ....7 Aspirate all blood that is possible (usually 10–20ml).
> 8 Remove the syringe and close the tap leaving the cannula *in situ*.

> If the needle tip impinges on the myocardium an injury pattern will appear on the ECG denoted by ST elevation or depression and widening of the QRS complex. In this event the needle should be withdrawn a few millimetres until the complex returns to a normal pattern.

Partial aortic rupture

Partial aortic rupture may occur as a result of blunt chest trauma or deceleration injury. The diagnosis is made as a result of suspicion in relation to the history of the injury. The clinical signs may be undramatic — modest hypotension and tachycardia with back pain.

Chest X-ray may show some or all of the following diagnostic features:
- Widened mediastinum.
- Obliteration of the aortic knob.
- Deviation of trachea and right main bronchus to the right.
- Deviation of the oesophagus to the right (marked by the nasogastric tube).
- Depression of the left main bronchus.

Suspicion of aortic rupture should be confirmed by an aortogram. Immediate surgical repair or grafting under cardiopulmonary bypass is required.

Diaphragmatic rupture

This injury may occur as a result of blunt trauma to the abdomen, deceleration injury or direct penetrating injury through the chest or abdomen. The condition is more common on the left.

The history of injury is important because the clinical signs may be unremarkable. The diagnostic features may include:
- Dyspnoea and tachypnoea.
- Cyanosis in severe cases.
- Pain radiating to the shoulder site.
- Bowel sounds audible in the thoracic cavity.

The diagnosis is confirmed by radiology. The chest X-ray may show a raised hemi-diaphragm and bowel

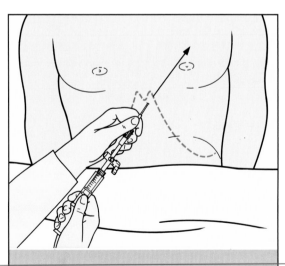

Fig. 3.26 Needle pericardiocentesis.

will be present in the thorax (possibly indicated by the nasogastric tube). Contrast radiography may show stomach herniating through the diaphragm. Surgical repair is required.

Tracheobronchial injury

Intrathoracic tracheal or bronchial injuries occur as a result of blunt trauma or deceleration injury. Major injuries are generally fatal.

In survivors the diagnostic features include:
- Dyspnoea and tachypnoea.
- Haemoptysis.
- Subcutaneous emphysema.
- Evidence of pneumothorax.
- A very large air leak through the chest drain.

The treatment consists of resuscitation using a double-lumen endobronchial tube to secure the airway and artificial ventilation, possibly using high frequency jet ventilation prior to direct surgical repair at thoracotomy.

Oesophageal injury

Oesophageal injury is rare. It may occur as a result of penetrating chest trauma or severe blunt trauma to the abdomen which forces air from the stomach into the oesophagus.

The clinical signs include:
- Severe retrosternal and back pain.
- Signs of pneumothorax on the left side.
- Haemothorax.
- Evidence of gastric contents in the chest drain.

Chest X-ray shows mediastinal emphysema and the injury site can be confirmed by a contrast swallow or oesophagoscopy. Surgical repair may be attempted if the diagnosis is made early.

THE ABDOMEN

Abdominal trauma is common and may arise as a result of blunt or penetrating injury.

Blunt injury

Blunt abdominal injury occurs commonly with motor accidents. Both occupants and pedestrians can be injured. Blunt injury generally causes splenic, liver or kidney rupture and shearing mesenteric lacerations.

Hollow viscus perforation may also occur. There may be no external evidence of injury.

Penetrating injury

Penetrating injury to abdominal organs can arise from entrance wounds in the limbs, buttocks and chest, as well as the abdomen. Stab injuries affect organs directly in their path. Bullets may follow a winding route due to tumble and rotation. Penetrating injury commonly involves the bowel, liver and kidney.

Severe haemorrhage is the commonest cause of death in the early stages after abdominal injury. Unfortunately the diagnoses of many cases of serious abdominal injury are still missed or made late, resulting in unnecessary fatalities. It is not important to make a precise diagnosis of the organs which are injured, but it is important to determine that an injury has occurred.

Examination and management

The examination of the patient with an abdominal injury should be systematic (Fig. 3.27) and integrated with the immediate management as clinical symptoms are detected.

Immediate management
- Clear the airway and support ventilation if required.
- Give oxygen therapy ($F_1O_2 \geq 0.85$).
- Establish two intravenous lines.
- Remove blood samples for cross matching, haematocrit, full blood count and amylase determination.
- Begin transfusion according to estimated blood loss.
- Pass a nasogastric tube (via the mouth if a cribriform plate fracture is suspected) and look for blood in gastric contents.
- Pass a urinary catheter if possible. Look for blood in the urine and measure the urine flow rate.
- If it is not possible to pass a urinary catheter introduce a suprapubic catheter when the bladder is full.
- When, and if, the patient's condition permits, X-ray the chest, pelvis, abdomen and spine. Look for chest pathology, fractures of ribs, spine and pelvis and free gas in the abdominal cavity.
- In cases of doubt perform a diagnostic peritoneal lavage.

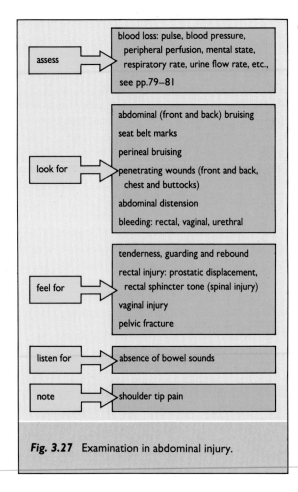

| assess | blood loss: pulse, blood pressure, peripheral perfusion, mental state, respiratory rate, urine flow rate, etc., see pp.79–81 |

look for	abdominal (front and back) bruising
	seat belt marks
	perineal bruising
	penetrating wounds (front and back, chest and buttocks)
	abdominal distension
	bleeding: rectal, vaginal, urethral

feel for	tenderness, guarding and rebound
	rectal injury: prostatic displacement, rectal sphincter tone (spinal injury)
	vaginal injury
	pelvic fracture

| listen for | absence of bowel sounds |

| note | shoulder tip pain |

Fig. 3.27 Examination in abdominal injury.

4 Make an incision 2cm long through the skin, fat, deep fascial layers and peritoneum.
5 Probe the wound with forceps to enter the abdominal cavity.
6 Insert a peritoneal catheter into the peritoneal cavity directing it towards the pelvis.
7 Aspirate from the catheter with a syringe.
8 If frank blood is not aspirated, instil 700ml Ringer lactate (10ml/kg) into the peritoneal cavity. Agitate the abdomen.
9 Siphon the fluid back after 10 minutes.
10 Examine the fluid.

A positive result is indicated by:
- Frank blood in the catheter.
- Evidence of 100,000 red cells/mm^3 .
- Evidence of 500 white cells/mm^3.

A negative result does not eliminate ruptured bowel, diaphragmatic rupture or retroperitoneal injury.

LIMB INJURIES

Limb injuries may be life-threatening if they are associated with unrecognized major blood loss. Losses of over 50 per cent of the blood volume may occur with major limb trauma and arterial injury. Severe crush injury is also potentially fatal. More often, however, poor early management leads to long-term disability.

In the examination of limbs (Fig. 3.29) the potentially injured part should always be compared with the uninjured part.

Diagnostic peritoneal lavage

Diagnostic peritoneal lavage is used to establish whether or not there is bleeding into the abdominal cavity (Fig. 3.28). It should only be used in cases of doubt.

The procedure is contraindicated in advanced pregnancy, extensive cirrhosis and in patients with pre-existing bleeding disorders.

Immediate management

The early management of limb injuries includes:
- Control of active bleeding by direct pressure.
- Replacement of lost blood volume.
- Traction splintage of lower limbs (check peripheral pulses and perfusion and sensation after traction has been applied).
- Pain relief.
- Tetanus immunization (if appropriate).

Technique
1 Decompress the stomach and bladder using a gastric tube and urinary catheter.
2 Prepare the skin over the lower abdomen with an antiseptic solution.
3 Inject local anaesthetic (lignocaine 1% with adrenaline) into the incision site in the midline of the distance between the umbilicus and symphysis pubis.

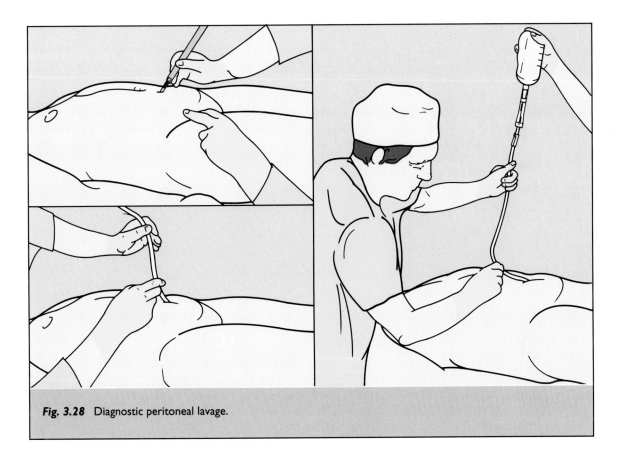

Fig. 3.28 Diagnostic peritoneal lavage.

• Broad spectrum antibiotics intravenously for contaminated wounds.

Early surgery will be required for:
• Persistent vascular or peripheral nerve compromise or injury (decompression and repair).
• Crush injury and the compartment syndrome (decompression and debridement).
• Open injuries (debridement and external fixation).
• Certain unstable fractures (internal or external fixation).

BURNS

Burns in the early stages threaten life by:
• Airway obstruction due to oedema formation within the respiratory tract.
• Inhalation of noxious gases.
• Hypovolaemia due to intravascular fluid loss.

Thermal injury to the respiratory tract

The onset of the full effects of thermal injury to the respiratory tract may be delayed for some hours. Once the airway is severely compromised recovery is very difficult. It is therefore essential to look for signs of inhalation injury early on and to secure the airway before serious impairment occurs.

The diagnostic features include:
• History of being confined in a burning environment.
• Confusion and mental impairment.
• Burns of nasal hair and eyebrows.
• Inflammation and oedema in the mouth and oropharynx.
• Carbon particles in the sputum.

Respiratory tract injury should be treated by tracheal intubation, oxygen therapy and ventilatory support according to clinical respiratory distress and arterial blood gas values.

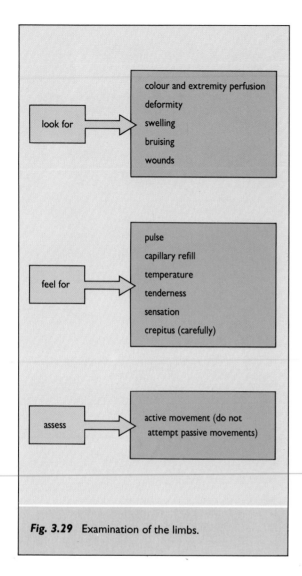

Fig. 3.29 Examination of the limbs.

Noxious gases

Carbon monoxide intoxication can be assumed in patients burned in a closed environment.

The diagnostic features may include:

• Headache.
• Nausea and vomiting.
• Confusion, drowsiness or unconsciousness.
• Cherry red skin coloration (an unreliable sign).

The diagnosis is confirmed by blood carbon monoxide levels. Carbon monoxide has a very high affinity for haemoglobin (240 times that of oxygen). Treatment consists of oxygen therapy, with an F_1O_2 of 1.0, to assist the breakdown of carboxyhaemoglobin. Ventilatory support may be required and serious cases may need to be treated in a hyperbaric chamber. Progress should be monitored by serial blood gas estimations.

Hypovolaemia

Hypovolaemia occurs approximately in proportion to the extent of the burn. This may be estimated using the "Rule of Nines".

Chest and abdomen – front	18%
Chest and abdomen – back	18%
Legs 18 x2	36%
Arms 9 x2	18%
Head	9%
Perineum	1%
Total	100%

In infants the head represents proportionately more than 9 per cent and the legs proportionately less than 18 per cent. The surface of one side of the patients own hand represents 1 per cent.

Volume replacement is based on the percentage of the surface area burned. Replacement should be by the intravenous route in all burns over 20 per cent. At least two intravenous cannulae should be inserted.

The replacement volume required should be assessed according to the urine flow rate and by arterial and central venous pressure measurements. Urinary flow rates of 30–50ml/h should be aimed for in adults (1ml/h in infants and children). As a rule, i.v. replacement volumes of 2–4ml/kg body weight per percentage burn are required in the first 24 hours. Half of this total should be given in the first eight hours and the remainder over 16 hours. These volume requirements are in addition to the patient's normal needs. One-third of the replacement volume should be with a colloid (e.g. a polygelatin or albumen solution) and the remainder with a crystalloid electrolyte solution (e.g. Ringer lactate). Blood will be required for most burns over 30 per cent. Hypertonic saline solutions may be used in the prehospital phase where difficult conditions present for i.v. cannulation as relatively small volumes are required for effective circulatory resuscitation.

In children where intravenous access may be very difficult interosseous screws may be placed on the anterior aspect of the upper tibia through which volume replacement (and drugs) may be given (Fig. 3.30)

Circumferential burns

Circumferential burns may constrict the peripheral circulation. The diagnostic features of impaired perfusion include:
• Peripheral cyanosis.
• Slow capillary refill.
• Absent peripheral pulses.
• Paraesthesia or loss of sensation.
Circumferential burns around the chest and neck may impair ventilation.
The treatment is to relieve the constriction by escharotomy.

Care of the burned surface
• Small burned areas (10 per cent) can be treated by the application of clean cold water immediately after burning. This reduces pain and the extent of thermal skin damage.
• Clothes contaminated with chemicals or burning plastic should be removed to stop the burning process and the burned surface irrigated in water to remove the contaminant.
• The burned surface should be covered with a loose plastic dressing (plastic bags for limbs) to minimize microbiological contamination.

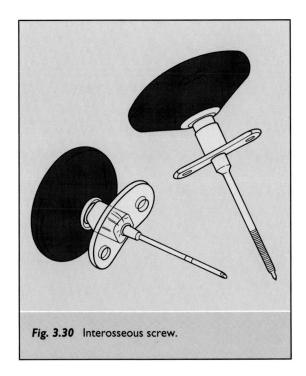

Fig. 3.30 Interosseous screw.

Electrical burns

Electrical burns may be more serious than they appear. Severe underlying muscle damage may occur, with myoglobinuria sufficient to cause renal failure.

Intravenous volume replacement should aim for high urinary flow rates (70–100ml/h) and should include mannitol, 25g initially and 12.5g intermittently to maintain a diuresis.

COLD INJURY AND HYPOTHERMIA

Local cold injury may be classified as freezing (frostbite) or non- freezing (trenchfoot).

Freezing injury

In freezing injury intracellular ice crystals have formed and the local microcirculation is occluded. The degree of injury depends on the depth of tissue damage. Examination may reveal:
• Hyperaemia and oedema without skin necrosis.
• Vesicle formation and partial skin necrosis.
• Full thickness skin necrosis.
• Necrosis of the skin and underlying tissues with gangrene formation.

Non-freezing injury

Non-freezing injury occurs in extremities exposed for some time to cold temperatures just above freezing point. Microvascular occlusion may develop and the affected part may appear black even though permanent tissue damage has not occurred.

Treatment
Patients with freezing and non-freezing injuries should be undressed, wrapped in warm blankets and given warm fluids by mouth. The extremity should be immersed in warm water at 40°C until the circulation returns to parts not irreversibly damaged (usually 30–60 minutes).

Hypothermia

Hypothermia commonly occurs as a result of immersion in water, even at modest temperatures (20°C), and after exposure to a cold environment with inactivity. Hypothermia is determined by measuring core (rectal or oesophageal) temperature with a low reading thermometer or thermistor probe.

Hypothermia is classified broadly according to core temperature:

• Mild (35–32°C).
• Moderate (32–30°C).
• Severe (<30°C).

The normal immediate physiological response to hypothermia is peripheral vasoconstriction which reduces heat loss. This is mediated by catecholamine release which also causes shivering to increase heat production. These responses disappear at core temperatures around 34–32°C (earlier in the elderly).

Effects of hypothermia

Hypothermia causes:

• Depression of consciousness.
• Depression of respiratory minute volume.
• Reduction in oxygen consumption.
• Depression of cardiac output, arterial pressure and pulse rate, with dysrrhythmias occurring below 33°C and ventricular fibrillation often developing at or below 30°C.

Some patients may continue to retain a very slow spontaneous heart beat, which is virtually undetectable clinically, down to temperatures of 20°C. This slight cardiac activity may be sufficient to satisfy the reduced cerebral oxygen requirements at such low temperatures and would explain the remarkable records of survival after immersion in cold water for periods of 45–60 minutes. Patients with a spontaneous but slow pulse should be handled very carefully and not given chest compressions as ventricular fibrillation may be precipitated.

Resuscitation of the hypothermic patient

Resuscitation of the hypothermic patient involves maintenance of the airway and support of ventilation and the circulation pending rewarming by active or passive measures (Fig. 3.31).

In all patients with severe hypothermia, attempts should be made to monitor arterial pressure through an arterial cannula. A close watch should be kept on the ECG because ventricular fibrillation can be precipitated during the rewarming process.

Patients with hypothermic cardiac arrest should be resuscitated with external chest compressions followed by open chest cardiac massage if cardiopulmonary bypass facilities with a heat exchanger are available. Defibrillation and the drugs used in cardiac arrest are not generally effective at core temperatures below 33°C.

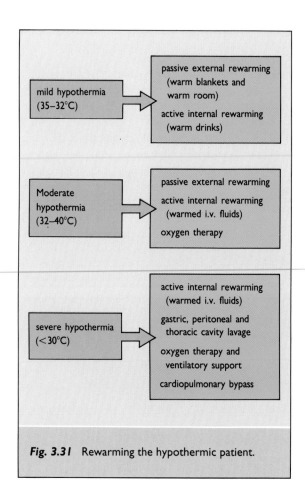

Fig. 3.31 Rewarming the hypothermic patient.

mild hypothermia (35–32°C)
→ passive external rewarming (warm blankets and warm room)
active internal rewarming (warm drinks)

Moderate hypothermia (32–40°C)
→ passive external rewarming
active internal rewarming (warmed i.v. fluids)
oxygen therapy

severe hypothermia (<30°C)
→ active internal rewarming (warmed i.v. fluids)
gastric, peritoneal and thoracic cavity lavage
oxygen therapy and ventilatory support
cardiopulmonary bypass

PAEDIATRIC RESUSCITATION

PAEDIATRIC RESUSCITATION

The basic life support of infants (under 1-year-old) (Fig. 4.1) and children (over 1-year-old) (Fig. 4.2) follows a similar format to that described for adults. Management of the airway and breathing take priority   in children; primary cardiac events are rare.

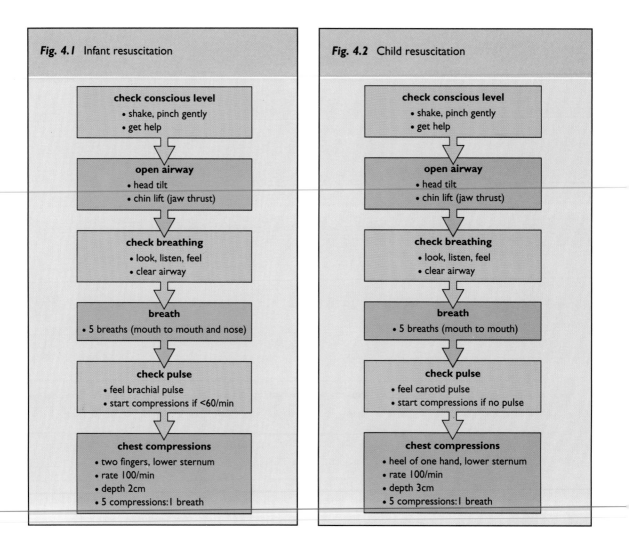

Fig. 4.1 Infant resuscitation

check conscious level
- shake, pinch gently
- get help

open airway
- head tilt
- chin lift (jaw thrust)

check breathing
- look, listen, feel
- clear airway

breath
- 5 breaths (mouth to mouth and nose)

check pulse
- feel brachial pulse
- start compressions if <60/min

chest compressions
- two fingers, lower sternum
- rate 100/min
- depth 2cm
- 5 compressions:1 breath

Fig. 4.2 Child resuscitation

check conscious level
- shake, pinch gently
- get help

open airway
- head tilt
- chin lift (jaw thrust)

check breathing
- look, listen, feel
- clear airway

breath
- 5 breaths (mouth to mouth)

check pulse
- feel carotid pulse
- start compressions if no pulse

chest compressions
- heel of one hand, lower sternum
- rate 100/min
- depth 3cm
- 5 compressions:1 breath

CAUSES OF CARDIAC ARREST

- Hypoxia
- Hypovolaemia (loss of blood or body fluids)
- Septicaemia
- Sudden Infant Death Syndrome
- Congenital heart disease

The first priority in children, therefore, must be to establish a patent airway and to restore breathing.

CLEARANCE AND MAINTENANCE OF THE AIRWAY USING BASIC LIFE SUPPORT

The child's airway is opened primarily by tilting the head backwards and supporting the mandible. If a clear airway is not obtained at the first attempt then repositioning should be tried. Careful alignment will produce a patent airway in the majority of patients.

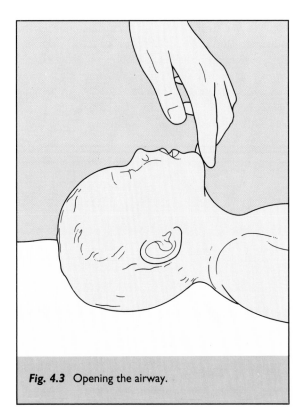

Fig. 4.3 Opening the airway.

Technique

1 Tilt the head backwards by pushing gently on the forehead.
2 Support and lift the mandible forwards using the tips of fingers on the bony tip of the chin (chin lift) (Fig. 4.3) or on the mandibular rami (jaw thrust). ●●●●●

- Do not overextend the baby's neck as this may kink and obstruct the trachea.
- Do not press on the soft tissues in the floor of the mouth as this may push the tongue into the airway.

●●●3 Where there are no teeth, it may be helpful to oppose the alveolar ridges to give some positional shape to the infant's airway.

Having attained an airway, careful observation and adjustments will be needed to maintain it.

As infants are obligatory nose breathers, it is vitally important to maintain clear nasal passages to ensure effective respiration in small children.

The Obstructed Airway

Causes of Obstruction
- Foreign material
- Infection
- Haemorrhage
- Tumours

Children will place a variety of foreign materials in their mouth many of which may cause an upper airway obstruction. The most common cause is regurgitated or vomited food. In any child whose upper airway is obstructed by foreign material, the obstruction should be cleared immediately by manual methods.

Haemorrhage from trauma to the head or neck may also cause airway obstruction; therefore, it is essential always to ensure that blood flows away from the airway and not into it. Tumours, although not necessarily associated with acute obstruction, can severely compromise the airway. Small increases in size of these tumours due to haemorrhage or oedema can result in sudden airway obstruction.

Manual methods of removing foreign material

Technique – finger sweeps
1 Open the mouth by pressure on the mandible and visualize the foreign body causing obstruction.
2 With a gloved finger, sweep or hook out the object causing the obstruction from the mouth.

Never use finger sweeps when the foreign objects cannot be seen. Blind finger probing may result in trauma, haemorrhage, oedema of the upper airway or further impaction of the foreign body.

Where the finger sweep has failed or the foreign body cannot be seen the airway may be cleared with back blows.

Technique – back blows
1 Place the child head down along the rescuer's thigh or arm (see Fig. 2.12).
2 Give a series of five blows on the middle of the back to give a forced expiration to expel the foreign material.

Abdominal thrusts

In older children abdominal thrusts may be an alternative method of generating an artificial cough to clear the airway.

Technique
1 Stand behind the victim and wrap the arms around the child just below the lower margin of the rib cage.
2 Clasp the hands tightly together and give a series of sharp upward thrusts, timed with expiration if discernable (see Fig. 2.13).
3. If the enforced expiration does not expel the offending obstruction, attempt to remove the obstruction with finger sweeps.

Obstructed Airway - Infection

Infectious diseases of the upper airway can cause serious and even fatal obstruction in small children.

Infectious causes of airway obstruction
• Croup
• Laryngotracheobronchitis
• Epiglottis

Stridor is the characteristic sign of impending problems. In most cases the child will be most comfortable sitting up and leaning forward. Humidified oxygen-enriched air should be given. In all serious cases expert help must be sought immediately. Further active intervention before such help is to hand may lead to a rapid worsening of the condition. Rather than waiting for deterioration to occur, the child should be transported to hospital so that the airway may be secured early under carefully administered inhalational anaesthesia with monitoring.

MAINTENANCE OF THE AIRWAY USING ADVANCED LIFE SUPPORT

Although the airway can be maintained without artificial aids in the majority of cases, some patients require further intervention for stability and control.

The oropharyngeal (Guedel) airway

The correct size will extend from the centre of the child's mouth to the angle of the jaw (Fig. 4.4). 'Size 0' is suitable for a six-month-old baby and a 'Size 1' for a 2-year-old child. Too small an airway will not overcome the obstruction caused by the tongue, whereas too large an airway may damage the posterior pharyngeal wall when it is inserted.

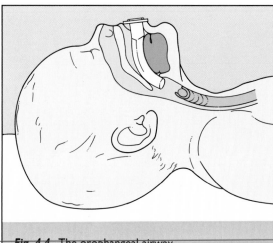

Fig. 4.4 The orophangeal airway.

If insertion of an oral airway does not result in a patent airway then it should be removed.

Nasopharyngeal airways

Although nasopharyngeal airways are not manufactured for children a tracheal tube of suitable diameter (4mm for a 6-month-old baby) cut to a short length and carefully secured can be used as a good substitute.

Laryngeal mask airway

The laryngeal mask airway has been successfully used in the management of known difficult airway problems in children and deserves further study.

> **Technique**
> The adult technique is described on pp.22–25. Two modification have been suggested for paediatric use.
>
> *1* Insert the laryngeal mask airway upside down and rotate it into position in the same way as advocated for the oropharyngeal airway.
> *2* Insert the laryngeal mask airway with the cuff partially inflated.

- Absence of breath sounds or inability to ventilate will require repositioning of the airway.
- Secure the airway firmly in place - accidental dislodgement can occur due to the relatively high position of the larynx.
- Posterior pharyngeal wall trauma has been exacerbated when using the laryngeal mask airway in children.
- The laryngeal mask airway may not protect against aspiration of gastric contents nor against the inhalation of secretions. The latter have been reported to accumulate and block the mask aperture. Regular suction should be used in such cases.

Tracheal intubation

Tracheal intubation is the only method of guaranteeing the airway. Intubation requires specific training on paediatric manikins to develop the particular skills to be used in infants.

Equipment for Paediatric Intubation

The equipment includes a laryngoscope with a straight blade, a selection of sizes of tracheal tubes with standard connectors, a flexible stylet, lubricating jelly, Magill's forceps, tape to secure the tube, scissors and suction apparatus.

Laryngoscope

Classically a straight laryngoscope blade is used – a size O or Seward, Miller, Robertshaw or Macintosh design is suitable (Fig. 4.5).

Tracheal tube

A straight sided uncuffed tracheal tube is recommended. The shouldered (Cole) tube should not be used as it may cause laryngeal injury. The tube should be fitted with a 15mm standard connector.

- to select the correct internal diameter (mm) use the formula: (age of child ÷ 4) + 4.
- to select the correct length (cm) use the formula: (age of child ÷ 2) + 12.

The technique of tracheal intubation is essentially the same as that used in adults. However, there are some significant differences in anatomy. The infant's

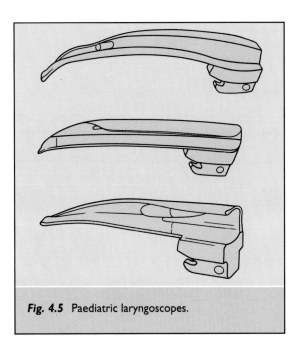

Fig. 4.5 Paediatric laryngoscopes.

larynx is located higher in the neck than in the adult, and the epiglottis is relatively large and floppy.

Technique

1 When using a straight blade laryngoscope, insert the blade beneath the epiglottis above the glottic opening (Fig. 4.6) and lift the long floppy epiglottis directly out of the way.

2 The narrowest diameter of the airway in the child is just below at the cricoid ring and not, as in the adult, the space between the vocal cords. Thus the size of tube must be carefully selected to slip easily between the cords and into the trachea (Fig. 4.7). Cuffed tubes are only used in sizes greater than 6mm diameter. Once in position there should be a small leak around the tube during positive pressure ventilation.

3 The trachea is relatively short and the tube must be carefully placed to avoid bronchial intubation. After positioning the tube, the chest must be auscultated to ensure bilateral and equal air entry.

4 A 15mm connector fixed to the end of the tracheal tube will attach directly to a self inflating resuscitation bag. In small children long connectors/adaptors should not be used as they will increase the dead space and reduce ventilatory efficiency.

Cricothyrotomy

Needle and surgical cricothyrotomy are emergency procedures which can be used to secure an airway when normal tracheal intubation cannot be achieved due to anatomical abnormality or maxillo-facial trauma.

Technique for needle cricothyrotomy

1 Introduce a 16G cannula over the needle percutaneously through the cricothyroid membrane and direct the cannula in a caudal direction.

2 Remove the needle and connect the cannula to the stem of a Y-piece connector.

3 Attach an oxygen supply at 8-10 l/min to one of the limbs on the Y.

4 Briefly occlude the other limb of the Y-piece until the chest rises. Expiration occurs by releasing the Y-piece occlusion until the chest has deflated.

Technique for surgical cricothyrotomy

1 Make a short horizontal incision (1cm) over the cricothyroid membrane.

2 Spread the skin and underlying structures apart with forceps and a retractor. The cricothyroid membrane is visualized.

3 Penetrate the cricothyroid membrane and insert and suture an appropriate sized tracheotomy tube in place.

Care must be taken not to cut the first intracheal ring as permanent airway damage may occur.

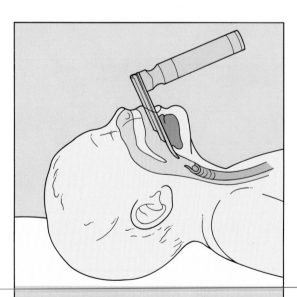

Fig. 4.6 Use of the laryngoscope in the infant.

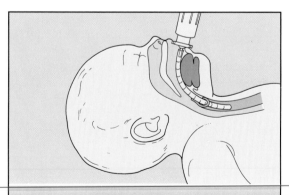

Fig. 4.7 Tracheal intubation.

BREATHING

As in adults breathing is assessed by:
- Looking for chest movement.
- Listening for air entry.
- Feeling for air movement.

See-saw abdominal movements indicate an obstructed airway. Inspiratory and expiratory stridor are often the first signs of infection causing airway closure. A sinister sign is a reduction in this stridor which may be interpreted as an apparent improvement in the airway but may in fact signal deterioration as less air is passing through the larynx as respiration fails.

Effective ventilation can be achieved by expired air resuscitation. In small children and babies this is usually by a mouth to mouth and nose technique.

Technique for mouth to mouth and nose method

1. Open the airway by pushing gently on the forehead to tilt the head backwards (Fig. 4.8).
2. Support and lift the mandible forwards using the tips of fingers on the chin.
3. Cover and seal the mouth and nose of the child with your mouth.
4. Blow into the child's mouth and nose. Stop blowing when the chest expands to the volume equivalent of a 'deep breath' (Fig. 4.9)
5. Allow the child to exhale passively.
6. Repeat this manoeuvre five times at a rate of one breath every three seconds. If difficulty is encountered the airway position should be readjusted and eight further attempts to ventilate made.

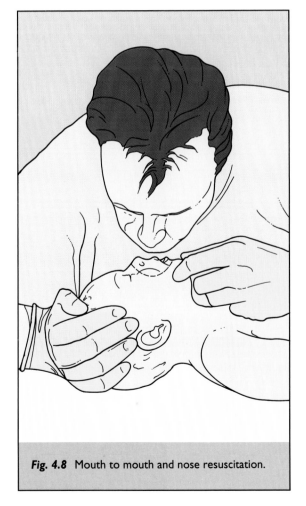

Fig. 4.8 Mouth to mouth and nose resuscitation.

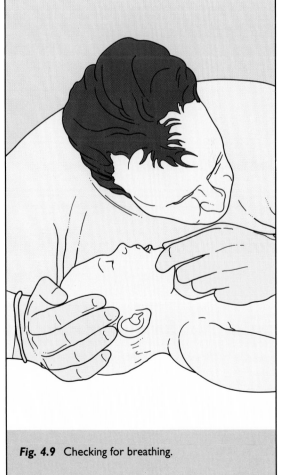

Fig. 4.9 Checking for breathing.

Self inflating bag/valve device

These devices are fully described on pp.37–39. The following additional points in relation to children should be noted.

- When using a self inflating bag/valve device, select a bag that can deliver 10–15ml/kg tidal volume (Fig. 4.10). The best choice is the mid-size bag 250–750ml.
- Paediatric self inflating bag/valve devices fitted with an oxygen reservoir will deliver up to 80 per cent inspired oxygen at an oxygen flow rate of 10 l/min.
- Many paediatric self inflating bag/valve devices are fitted with pressure limiting valves. These prevent barotrauma by blowing off at 35–45cmH20. In resuscitation these valves should be inactivated.
- A circular face mask is recommended when resuscitating small children.

Barotrauma to the lungs with resultant pneumothorax can occur during paediatric resuscitation. A sudden change in lung compliance, an alteration in ventilation charcteristics, hypoxia or circulatory failure should alert the rescuer to this possibility.

Oxygen powered resuscitators

These devices are not recommended for resuscitation in babies and small children because the appropriate tidal volumes may be difficult to select and high airway pressures may develop.

CIRCULATION

There are certain special aspects of resuscitation of the circulation in infants and small children.

Palpable pulses

Infants under one-year of age have relatively short chubby necks making palpation of the carotid pulse difficult. In this age group the brachial pulse is palpated (Fig. 4.11). In older children use the carotid pulse (see Fig. 2.58).

Bradycardia

A heart rate below 60 beats/min in infants under one year of age indicates the need for circulatory support. Bradycardia in this age group is almost as detrimental as asystole. Chest compressions and advanced circulatory support must be started when a severe bradycardia occurs. To wait for asystole may result in severe brain and major organ damage.

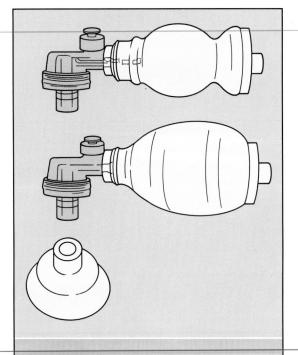

Fig. 4.10 Self inflating bags and paediatric mask.

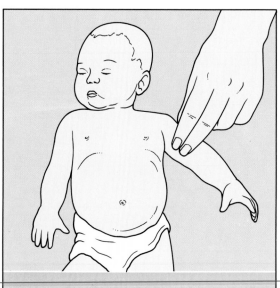

Fig. 4.11 Checking for a pulse.

External Chest Compressions

External chest compression is the basic method of maintaining the child's circulation during bradycardia or asystole For the mechanism of action see pp.42–46.

> ### Technique (infants under one year)
> 1 Place the infant supine on a firm surface.
> 2 Imagine a line between the nipples (Fig. 4.12).
> 3 Place the middle three fingers of one hand along the sternum below this line.
> 4 Lift the upper finger on the sternum. Use the lower two fingers to compress the sternum 2cm at a rate of 100/min.

> ### Technique (children over one year)
> 1 Place the child supine on a firm surface.
> 2 Place two fingers on the xiphisternum and place the heel of the other hand above, on the sternum in the midline (Fig. 4.13).
> 3 Compress the sternum 3cm with the heal of one hand at a rate of 100/min.

In children over eight years of age the two–handed adult technique should be used.

Co-ordination of Ventilation and Chest Compressions

In infants and children under eight years give five compressions followed by one breath (compression rate 100/min, respirations 20/min). When the adult two-handed compression is used perform 15 compressions to two breaths.

ADVANCED CIRCULATORY SUPPORT

Restoration of the Spontaneous Heartbeat

As with adults, treatment will depend on the nature of the arrest displayed on the electrocardiogram (ECG). The ECG is best recorded in infants by using self adhesive electrodes. Electrodes are placed above the left and right nipples and on the left leg. Defibrillator paddle electrodes can be used to monitor the ECG but, because of their relatively large size, give a poor contact area. The contact area can be improved by using a front to back position, turning the child on its side, but this requires the temporary cessation of chest compressions during the diagnostic phase.

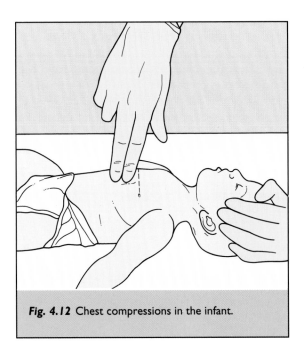

Fig. 4.12 Chest compressions in the infant.

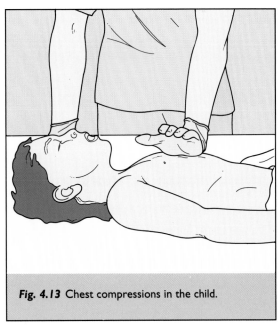

Fig. 4.13 Chest compressions in the child.

ECG Rhythms

Bradycardia and asystole

A slow heart rate or asystole is the commonest cause of circulatory failure in infants and small children.

A bradycardia is defined as a rate below 60 beats/min for infants under one year-old and below 40 beats/min when over one-year-old.

Slow or absent rhythms are best treated by ensuring good ventilation and oxygenation, together with effective chest compressions. As most such incidents in small infants are related to airway and breathing problems, this may be all that is necessary to restore an adequate circulation. Should the child not respond then the adult advanced life support protocol using scaled-down doses of adrenaline and atropine should be followed (see pp.59–60).

Ventricular fibrillation

This rhythm is relatively uncommon in children and is usually only seen as the terminal stage of a cardiac arrest. Treatment should follow the adult protocols but with the following modifications:

■ **DEFIBRILATOR PADDLE SIZE**

Select the largest defibrillator paddle size that provides good skin contact and allows adequate paddle separation. Choosing the largest size ensures low transthoracic impedance and improves the chance of defibrillation. As a rough guide use 4.5cm diameter paddles for infants and 8.0cm or 13cm paddles for older children. Where a small child presents for defibrillation and only large paddles are available, turn the child on its side and defibrillate from front to back.

■ **ENERGY DOSE**

The energy dose required to defibrillate infants has not been scientifically evaluated for the clinical environment. Current recommendations are 2J/kg, doubling this dose if the initial attempts are unsuccessful. It is recognized that the calculated energy dose will only approximate to that available from the defibrillator, especially if the machine used will only charge to preset levels (25, 50, 100J).

If initial defibrillation is unsuccessful then adult advanced life support protocols using modified drug doses should be followed.

Electromechanical dissociation (EMD)

EMD is usually seen in children following trauma. Hypovolaemia, cardiac tamponade and tension pneumothorax are the most common causes. As in adults it is important to diagnose and treat the underlying cause, while maintaining adequate ventilation and oxygenation throughout.

Vascular Access

Obtaining vascular access in a small infant is probably the most difficult of the advanced procedures and yet it is one of the most important. It is essential to establish reliable vascular access early in the protocol to restore depleted circulating blood volume and to administer medications.

In children central cannulation does provide more direct access for drug administration but is a highly skilled technique which may not be available to many rescuers. Peripheral venous cannulation does have the disadvantage of being distant from the central circulation but is a relatively straightforward technique, and may be the preferred route. The intraosseous and endobronchial routes should also be considered.

Peripheral route

These same sites are available in children as in adults. The cephalic, median, basilic and median antecubital veins in the forearm, however, are difficult to locate in chubby babies. In the lower extremity saphenous veins and veins comprising the dorsal arch in the foot can be used (Fig. 4.14). The cutdown technique for the long saphenous vein as it passes anterior to the medial malleolus has been described previously (see pp.93–94). It may be a particularly valuable alternative in children over the age of three. Scalp veins are small and difficult to maintain during resuscitation, but they may be considered for intravenous access when stability has been achieved.

Central route

The techniques of central venous access have been described on pp.90–94 The most common access sites in children are the internal and external jugular vein, the subclavian vein and the femoral vein. It is necessary to develop and maintain special skills when applying these techniques in small children.

Intraosseous route

The intraosseous route is particularly valuable in children. Crystalloid and colloid fluid have been safely replaced and drugs such as catecholamines, calcium, digitalis, heparin, lignocaine, atropine, sodium bicarbonate and antibiotics have also been successfully infused. A 0.6 per cent incidence of osteomyelitis was found in children receiving intraosseous infusions of two days duration.

Technique

1 Select a site on the anterior aspect of the tibia, 1–3cm below the tibial tuberosity. Do not use a limb which has a proximal fracture or compromised vascular supply.
2 Prepare the skin over the site with antiseptic solution.
3 Direct a paediatric intraosseous needle perpendicularly into the tibia until it is sited in the marrow cavity.
4 Entry into the marrow cavity occurs when a loss of resistance to needle insertion is felt; marrow can be aspirated through the needle and fluid can be injected without subcutaneous infiltration (Fig. 4.15). ⬛⬛⬛⬛⬛

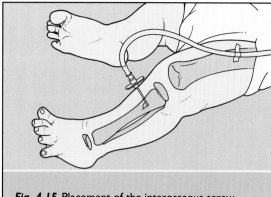

Fig. 4.15 Placement of the interosseous screw.

- Care must be taken to insert the needle at least 1cm below the tibial tuberosity to avoid damaging the epiphyseal growth plate.
- Tibial fracture has been reported after distal needle insertion.

⬛⬛⬛⬛5 Fluid infusion or drug administration may be achieved either by direct injection or pressure infusion through the needle into the marrow cavity.
6 Intraosseous infusion should be regarded as a short term vascular access and should be replaced by formal, direct intravascular access when possible.

Endobronchial route

This is described on p.63. In the early stages of resuscitation, this may be the only access available for the essential resuscitation drugs such as adrenaline. It should only be used in these very early stages of resuscitation as the absorption of drugs may be unreliable for this route. Doses should be 2–3 times that advocated for the intravenous route.

Intravenous Fluid Administration

A child's blood volume is 80–90ml/kg. Fluid administration should aim to restore the circulating blood volume and although authorities vary as to the pre-

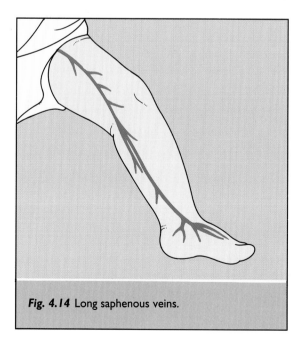

Fig. 4.14 Long saphenous veins.

119

cise volumes recommended, it is generally agreed that a crystalloid bolus of 20ml/kg should be given to treat hypovolaemia shock initially. This can be repeated up to three times (a maximum of 60ml/kg); 10–20ml/kg boluses of colloid (plasma or blood) can be given if the initial therapy is unsuccessful. The plasma substitutes, polygelatines and hetastarch can be used instead of plasma. Early fluid therapy is important in all forms of shock or circulatory collapse as children deteriorate rapidly with a low circulating blood volume.

> Not all the commercial products used in adults are licensed for use in children.

Drug Therapy

Drugs are best administered intravenously. although the intraosseous route is now considered as an early alternative when intravenous access is difficult. Endotracheal drug administration is not usually recommended in children because of the relatively large volumes required.

Drugs dosages are calculated from the body weight of the child.

Approximations for body weights

> Infants double their birth weight in five months
> Infants treble their birth weight in one year
> Aged 1–9 years weight (kg) = (age + 4) x 2
> Aged 7–12 years weight (kg) = age x 3

In the emergency situation the weight of a child may not always be immediately available. Guessing weight has been proven to be notoriously inaccurate. There are two systems of estimating weight from the child's height or length. Both methods are certainly better than guessing and their adoption may improve the management of resuscitation in children:-

The Oakley chart

This chart relates height to weight and to age (Fig. 4.16). Having obtained any of these parameters the size and length of the tracheal tube and the correct doses of drugs can be read off the chart.

The Broselaw measuring tape

This is a tape measure which when laid alongside the child will indicate the resuscitation equipment and drugs in the appropriate section and colour corresponding to the length of the child (Fig. 4.17).

Core Temperature

It is important to maintain as best possible the child's temperature during resuscitation. Unnecessary exposure should be avoided. Heating and humidifying inspired gases, warming intravenous fluids and the use of heat retaining blankets will reduce hypothermia during resuscitation.

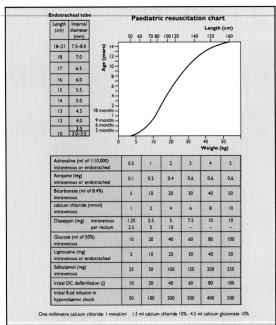

Fig. 4.16 The Oakley chart. (Reproduced by kind permission of Dr Peter Oakley and The British Medical Journal.)

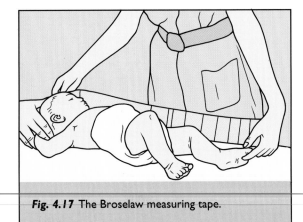

Fig. 4.17 The Broselaw measuring tape.

PAIN RELIEF

PAIN RELIEF

INTRODUCTION

Analgesia is a most important part of treatment both in relation to trauma and to the exquisite pain of myocardial infarction. Too often, however, pain relief is omitted or given in inadequate doses because of fears of side-effects from some of the agents in common use. These side-effects are often less profound in patients with severe pain than they are in those who are the subject of drug trials who may be relatively free from noxious stimuli.

Although the perfect analgesic is still awaited, much can be done with the agents currently available if they are properly used to exploit their beneficial properties.

THE PATHOPHYSIOLOGICAL RESPONSE TO PAIN

Although there is a clear indication to relieve pain purely on compassionate grounds, there is also a good reason for analgesia based on the pathophysiological response to pain.

Pain produces an outburst of sympathetic activity and catecholamine release which enhances vasoconstriction and tachycardia, which in turn reduces tissue perfusion and increases myocardial oxygen requirements. The reduction in tissue perfusion may further jeopardize the microcirculation in hypovolaemic and cardiogenic shock and extend the zone of infarction in myocardial ischaemia (Fig. 5.1).

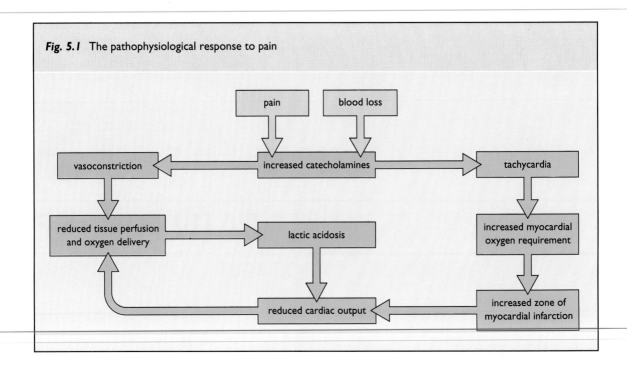

Fig. 5.1 The pathophysiological response to pain

ANALGESIC AGENTS

Features of the ideal analgesic in the emergency situation

The ideal analgesic in the emergency situation should have the following features:
- Powerful in action.
- Rapid onset.
- Speedy recovery.
- Not depressant to the cardiorespiratory system.
- Free of unwanted side-effects.
- Available for safe and easy use by non-physicians.
- Non-addictive.
- Easily portable.

The features of the ideal analgesic must be compared with the properties of the available agents.

Available agents

The available agents for use in the emergency situation include:
- Nitrous oxide/oxygen mixtures.
- The opiates: morphine, diamorphine, nalbuphine, buprenorphine etc.
- Ketamine.
- Non-steriodal analgesics (e.g. ketorolac, diclofenac)
- Local anaesthetic agents.

Nitrous oxide/oxygen mixture

Inhaled 50% nitrous oxide and oxygen is a powerful analgesic, equating to 10mg of morphine in the normal adult. The mixture is available in a single cylinder and is known as Entonox. It is self-administered by the patient, who inspires the gas mixture from a mask or mouthpiece. The inhalational apparatus incorporates a demand valve which ensures that no gas flows unless a negative pressure is generated by the patient inspiring while making a gas-tight seal between the mask and his face (Fig. 5.2). To do this the patient must be conscious and cooperative. The arrangement thus incorporates a clear fail-safe system which prevents further inhalation if the patient should become drowsy or unconscious.

Entonox has the following valuable features:
- Rapid onset (2 minutes).
- Speedy recovery once inhalation stops (2 minutes).
- Non-depressant to the cardiorespiratory system.
- No side-effects except drowsiness.

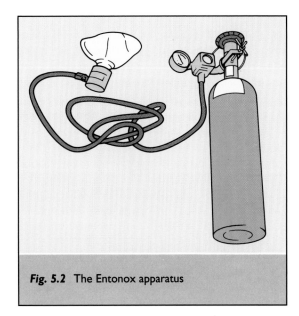

Fig. 5.2 The Entonox apparatus

- The apparatus is reasonably portable depending on cylinder size.
- Administration can be supervised safely by non-physicians.
- The administration ensures an F_1O_2 of 0.5.

There are a few contraindications:
- Absolute contraindications: pneumothorax, the bends, acute gastric dilation.
- Relative contraindications: the uncooperative and confused, maxillofacial injury, severe head injury.

Entonox has been shown to provide good pain relief in 66 per cent of all patients, moderate pain relief in a further 30 per cent and poor pain relief in only 3–4 per cent.

The opiates

The opiates are given parenterally by the intravenous route in small increments titrated against the patient's response. The intramuscular route is not suitable in the majority of emergency situations because of unreliable uptake from muscle which is poorly perfused in hypovolaemia and cardiogenic shock.

■ **THE NATURAL ALKALOIDS**

Diamorphine is generally agreed to be the most potent and effective analgesic, particularly in patients suffering from acute myocardial infarction. However, it is not generally available in all countries of the world. Diamorphine is given in 2.5mg increments intravenously.

Morphine is universally available and is effective in the majority of patients in 5mg increments intravenously. Morphine and diamorphine are more effective agents than the synthetic opiates. They do, however, have a number of unfortunate side-effects:

- In excessive dosage they cause respiratory and cardiovascular depression and depression of the laryngeal reflexes. This depression is less pronounced in patients with severe pain. The elderly, those with chest injuries and chronic obstructive airways disease, and patients in hypovolaemic and cardiogenic shock are particularly susceptible. Opiates should not be given to patients with major head injuries.
- They cause nausea and vomiting particularly if the patient is moved (e.g. in an ambulance or helicopter).
- They require administration by the intravenous route.
- They are addictive, and prescription is strictly controlled for issue to individual patients only by a physician.
- The duration of action is 30–60 minutes. The action can be reversed using naloxone 0.2–0.4mg intravenously.

■ THE SYNTHETIC OPIATES

Many synthetic opiates have been introduced into clinical practice but none have surpassed diamorphine and morphine in the emergency situation. Two agents have found a limited place — nalbuphine and buprenorphine. While not as potent as the natural products, and producing similar undesirable side-effects, they have some points in their favour:

- Depression of respiration is limited compared with diamorphine and morphine.
- Addiction to these synthetic opiates is not considered likely and they are not subject to the stringent regulations that apply to morphine and diamorphine.

Buprenorphine (0.4mg) may be administered by the sublingual route which obviates the need for intravenous cannulation. It is rapidly absorbed (5 minutes) from this site.

Nalbuphine is given in 5–10mg increments intravenously, and is the preferred agent of the two.

Ketamine

Ketamine is generally used as an anaesthetic agent but in smaller doses (0.25–0.5mg/kg) is an effective analgesic. Its principal advantage over the opiates is that it does not cause depression of the cardiovascular system, and interference with the laryngeal reflexes and respiration is minimal. Its principal clinical use has been in the prehospital situation and particularly in major disasters. Ketamine can be given by the intramuscular as well as the intravenous route and this may be valuable in the trapped or severely burned patient, when venous access cannot always be secured.

The main undesirable side-effect associated with ketamine is a high index of unpleasant dreams which cause considerable distress when they are recalled afterwards. These dreams occur particularly in the 15–45 age group. The incidence of dreams is however dose-related and is low when the drug is given in analgesic rather than anaesthetic doses. The dreams can be counteracted by the benzodiazepines (e.g. midazolam 5mg or Diazemuls 10mg).

Non-steroidal analgesics

These agents are suitable for moderate pain only when given alone. However they are remarkably free from cardiorespiratory depressant side-effects and may enable opiate dosage to be reduced in patients with severe pain.

Local anaesthesia

Local anaesthetic techniques are rarely appropriate for the relief of pain associated with the early phases of trauma. Two techniques are however of value:
- Intercostal nerve block.
- Femoral nerve block.

■ INTERCOSTAL NERVE BLOCK

Intercostal block is used for patients with fractured ribs in whom the pain is interfering with respiration (Fig. 5.3). It is particularly useful in patients with chronic obstructive airways disease. The intercostal block can later be replaced with thoracic epidural analgesia.

Technique
1 Identify the fractured ribs.
2 Prepare the skin in the posterior axillary line at the appropriate level with an antiseptic solution. ■ ■ ■ ■ ■ ■

3 Using 3–4ml of 1 per cent lignocaine with adrenaline for each space, infiltrate the skin, subcutaneous tissue and the intercostal space just beneath the affected ribs in the posterior axillary line. Also inject the spaces one above and one below the fractured levels. Note that the intercostal nerves run in the groove beneath the lower border of each rib.

The total dose of lignocaine must not exceed 200g of lignocaine in the normal adult (3mg/kg).

■ **FEMORAL NERVE BLOCK**

Femoral nerve block in the groin is most valuable in relieving the pain arising from a fractured shaft of femur (Fig. 5.4).

Technique

1 Prepare the skin in the groin with an antiseptic solution.
2 Identify the pulsation of the femoral artery. The femoral nerve lies 1cm lateral to the artery.
3 Infiltrate this region to a depth of 1–3cm (depending on the patient's obesity) with 5–10ml of lignocaine with adrenaline.

The benzodiazepines

The benzodiazepines are not analgesics in their own right. However, in the emergency situation they may be able to reduce the anxiety and distress so often associated with the pain of myocardial infarction or injury and thus reduce the amount of analgesic required. The benzodiazepines are not associated with cardiorespiratory depression or nausea and vomiting, so these side-effects may be avoided by reducing the total dose of the opiate.

Fig. 5.3 Intercostal nerve block

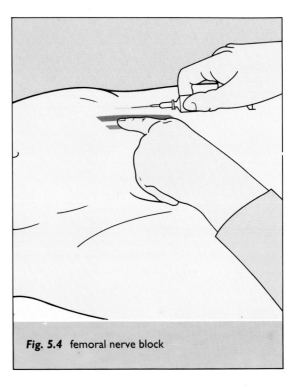

Fig. 5.4 femoral nerve block

A PLAN FOR THE MANAGEMENT OF PAIN

Using the available agents either singly or, if necessary, in combination, pain can be relieved in the majority of patients without serious uncontrollable side-effects developing.

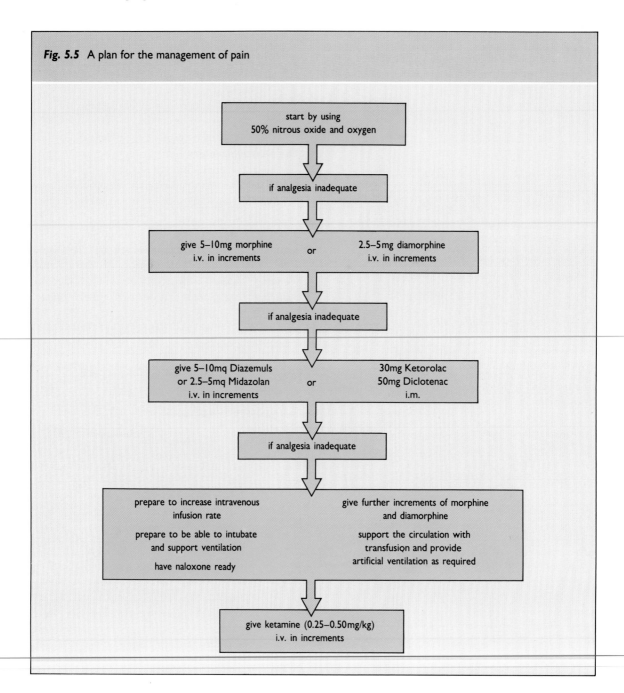

Fig. 5.5 A plan for the management of pain

start by using
50% nitrous oxide and oxygen

if analgesia inadequate

give 5–10mg morphine
i.v. in increments
or
2.5–5mg diamorphine
i.v. in increments

if analgesia inadequate

give 5–10mq Diazemuls
or 2.5–5mq Midazolan
i.v. in increments
or
30mg Ketorolac
50mg Diclotenac
i.m.

if analgesia inadequate

prepare to increase intravenous
infusion rate

prepare to be able to intubate
and support ventilation

have naloxone ready

give further increments of morphine
and diamorphine

support the circulation with
transfusion and provide
artificial ventilation as required

give ketamine (0.25–0.50mg/kg)
i.v. in increments

TRAINING REQUIREMENTS

TRAINING REQUIREMENTS

Figures 6.1 and 6.2 offer suggestions as to who should be taught the various skills involved in resuscitation. Clearly the situation will vary from locality to locality, with national traditions and, most importantly, with staffing levels in hospitals.

There is, however, little doubt that all doctors should be capable of managing a cardiac arrest, including the use of defibrillator and venous cannulation. Any nurse deemed capable of being responsible for patients in a ward should be capable of defibrillation. All doctors should be able to undertake a rapid assessment of the severely injured patient, control life-threatening airway and ventilation problems, and establish venous access and fluid replacement.

Fig. 6.1 Cardiac life support: who should be taught what?	lay public	rescue services	ambulance service	student nurse	RGN/RN	ward sister/head nurse	senior nurse in acute unit	medical student	houseman/intern	SHO/registrar/resident	consultant/staff	family doctor	military doctor
assessment	✓	✓	✓	✓	✓	✓	✓	✓	✓	✓	✓	✓	✓
basic airway control	✓	✓	✓	✓	✓	✓	✓	✓	✓	✓	✓	✓	✓
EAR	✓	✓	✓	✓	✓	✓	✓	✓	✓	✓	✓	✓	✓
ECC	✓	✓	✓	✓	✓	✓	✓	✓	✓	✓	✓	✓	✓
ACD	✓	✓	✓	✓	✓	✓	✓	✓	✓	✓	✓	✓	✓
oral airway	×	×	✓	✓	✓	✓	✓	✓	✓	✓	✓	✓	✓
laryngeal mask	×	×	✓	✓	✓	✓	✓	✓	✓	✓	✓	✓	✓
ETT	×	×	✓	×	×	×	✓	?	?	✓	✓	?	✓
cricothyrotomy	×	×	×	×	×	×	×	×	✓	✓	✓	✓	✓
mouth to mask	✓	✓	✓	✓	✓	✓	✓	✓	✓	✓	✓	✓	✓
self-inflating bag	×	×	✓	×	✓	✓	✓	?	?	✓	✓	?	✓
automatic resuscitator	×	?	✓	×	✓	✓	✓	✓	✓	✓	✓	✓	✓
ECG interpretation	×	×	✓	✓	✓	✓	✓	✓	✓	✓	✓	✓	✓
defibrillation: automatic	×	✓	✓	✓	✓	✓	✓	✓	✓	✓	✓	✓	✓
defibrillation: manual	×	×	✓	×	✓	✓	✓	✓	✓	✓	✓	✓	✓
peripheral i.v.	×	×	✓	×	✓	✓	✓	✓	✓	✓	✓	✓	✓
central i.v.	×	×	?	×	×	×	?	✓	✓	✓	✓	?	✓
cardiac puncture	×	×	×	×	×	×	×	✓	✓	✓	✓	✓	✓
arterial cannula	×	×	×	×	×	×	×	?	✓	✓	✓	×	?
atropine, lignocaine, adrenaline	×	×	✓	×	×	✓	✓	✓	✓	✓	✓	✓	✓
other drugs	×	×	×	×	×	×	×	✓	✓	✓	✓	?	?
open chest cardiac massage	×	×	×	×	×	×	×	×	×	✓	✓	×	✓
thrombolytic therapy	×	×	?	×	×	×	×	✓	✓	✓	✓	✓	?
Entonox	×	✓	✓	✓	✓	✓	✓	✓	✓	✓	✓	✓	✓
opiates	×	×	?	×	×	✓	✓	✓	✓	✓	✓	✓	✓

Fig. 6.2 Trauma life support: who should be taught what?

	lay public	rescue services	ambulance service	student nurse	RGN/RN	ward sister/head nurse	senior nurse in acute unit	medical student	houseman/intern	SHO/registrar/resident	consultant/staff	family doctor	military doctor
assessment: primary	✓	✓	✓	✓	✓	✓	✓	✓	✓	✓	✓	✓	✓
assessment: secondary	×	×	✓	×	?	✓	✓	✓	✓	✓	✓	✓	✓
control of spine	✓	✓	✓	✓	✓	✓	✓	✓	✓	✓	✓	✓	✓
basic airway control	✓	✓	✓	✓	✓	✓	✓	✓	✓	✓	✓	✓	✓
EAR	✓	✓	✓	✓	✓	✓	✓	✓	✓	✓	✓	✓	✓
ECC	✓	✓	✓	✓	✓	✓	✓	✓	✓	✓	✓	✓	✓
oral airway	×	×	✓	✓	✓	✓	✓	✓	✓	✓	✓	✓	✓
laryngeal mask	×	×	✓	✓	✓	✓	✓	✓	✓	✓	✓	✓	✓
ETT	×	×	✓	×	×	×	✓	?	?	✓	✓	✓	✓
cricothyrotomy	×	×	×	×	×	×	×	×	✓	✓	✓	✓	✓
mouth to mask	✓	✓	✓	✓	✓	✓	✓	✓	✓	✓	✓	✓	✓
self-inflating bag	×	×	✓	?	?	✓	✓	?	?	✓	✓	?	✓
automatic resuscitator	×	?	✓	×	✓	✓	✓	✓	✓	✓	✓	✓	✓
ECG interpretation	×	×	✓	✓	✓	✓	✓	✓	✓	✓	✓	✓	✓
defibrillation: automatic	×	✓	✓	✓	✓	✓	✓	✓	✓	✓	✓	✓	✓
defibrillation: manual	×	×	✓	×	✓	✓	✓	✓	✓	✓	✓	✓	✓
control of haemorrhage	✓	✓	✓	✓	✓	✓	✓	✓	✓	✓	✓	✓	✓
MAST	×	×	✓	×	×	×	✓	✓	✓	✓	✓	✓	✓
peripheral i.v.	×	×	✓	×	✓	✓	✓	✓	✓	✓	✓	✓	✓
central i.v.	×	×	?	×	×	×	?	✓	✓	✓	✓	?	✓
cut down i.v.	×	×	×	×	×	×	×	✓	✓	✓	✓	✓	✓
arterial cannula	×	×	×	×	×	×	×	?	✓	✓	✓	×	×
needle thoracostomy	×	×	✓	×	×	✓	✓	✓	✓	✓	✓	✓	✓
chest drain	×	×	×	×	×	×	×	✓	✓	✓	✓	×	✓
peritoneal lavage	×	×	×	×	×	×	×	×	×	✓	✓	×	✓
pericardiocentasis	×	×	×	×	×	×	×	✓	✓	✓	✓	✓	✓
open chest cardiac massage	×	×	×	×	×	×	×	×	×	✓	✓	×	✓
Entonox	×	✓	✓	✓	✓	✓	✓	✓	✓	✓	✓	✓	✓
opiates	×	×	?	×	×	✓	✓	✓	✓	✓	✓	✓	✓
ketamine	×	×	×	×	×	×	×	✓	✓	✓	✓	×	✓
local anaesthesia	×	×	×	×	×	×	×	✓	✓	✓	✓	✓	✓

FURTHER READING

1. Recommended Guidelines for Uniform Reporting of Data from Cardiac Arrest. The Utstein Style prepared by a Task Force of representatives from the American Heart Association, European Resuscitation Council, Heart and Stroke Foundation of Canada and the Australian Resuscitation Council. - Circulation 1991.

2. American College of Surgeons. *Advanced Trauma Life Support for Physicians.* Chicago: American College of Surgeons (55 East Erie Street, Chicago, Illinois 60611, USA), 1992.

3. American Heart Foundation. *Advanced Cardiac Life Support Manual.* Dallas: American Heart Foundation (7320 Greenville Avenue, Dallas, Texas 75231, USA), 1992.

4. American Heart Association. American Heart Association 1985 National Conference Standards and Guidelines for Cardiopulmonary Resuscitation (CPR) and Emergency Cardiac Care (ECC). *JAMA* 1992;**255**(Suppl).

5. Australian Resuscitation Council. *Policy Statements of the Australian Resuscitation Council.* Sydney: Australian Resuscitation Council.

6. European Resuscitation Council. Guidelines for Basic and Advanced Lift Support (1992) *Resuscitation.* 1992;**24**(2):103–123.

7. Resuscitation Council UK. *Basic and Advanced Life Support Guidelines of the Resuscitation Council UK, 1989.* London: Resuscitation Council UK (Department of Anaesthesia, Hammersmith Hospital, Ducane Road, London), 1989.

8. Resuscitation Council UK. *Resuscitation for the Citizen.* London: Resuscitation Council UK (Department of Anaesthesia, Hammersmith Hospital, Ducane Road, London), 1989.

9. Royal College of Physicians. *Report of the Royal College of Physicians on Cardiopulmonary Resuscitation, 1987.* London: Royal College of Physicians (Regent's Park, London), 1987.

10. Royal College of Surgeons. *Report of the Working Party of the Royal College of Surgeons on the Management of Patients with Major Injuries.* London: Royal College of Surgeons of England (Lincoln's Inn Fields, London), 1988.

11. Baskett PJF, ed. *Cardiopulmonary Resuscitation.* Amsterdam: Elsevier, 1989.

12. Baskett PJF. Ethics in resuscitation. *Resuscitation* 1993;**25**(1):1–8.

13. Baskett PJF, Weller RM, eds. *Medicine for Disasters.* London: Butterworths (John Wright), 1988.

14. Benimoff JL, ed. *Clinical Procedures in Anesthesia and Intensive Care.* Philadelphia, JB Lippincott, 1992.

15. Bossaert L, Koster R. Defibrillation: methods and strategies. *Resuscitation.* 1992;**24**(2):211–226.

16. Caroline NL. *Ambulance Calls. Review Problems in Emergency Care.* Boston, MA: Little Brown & Co, 1987.

17. Caroline NL. *Emergency Care in the Streets.* Boston, MA: Little Brown & Co, 1987.

18. Caroline NL. *Emergency Medical Treatment.* Boston, MA: Little Brown & Co, 1987.

19. Cummins RO, Ornato JP, Theis WH, Pepe PE. *Improving Survival from Sudden Arrest – The Chain of Survival Concept.* Office of Scientific Affairs, American Heart Association, Dallas, 1991.

20. Delooz HH, Mullie A, Dick WF, *et. al*. Forms for registration of CPR effects and outcome, respectively for out-of-hospital cardiac arrest. *Resuscitation.* 1992;**24**(2):155–166.

21. Eisenberg MS, Bergner L, Hallstrom AP. *Sudden Death in the Community.* New York: Praeger, 1984.

22. Evans TR, ed. *ABC of Resuscitation,* 2nd edition. London: British Medical Journal, 1988.

23. Grande CM, ed. *Textbook of Trauma Anaesthesia and Critical Care.* Philadelphia: Mosby Year Book, 1992.

24. Haynes SA, Robertson C. CPR – drug delivery routes and systems. *Resuscitation* 1992;**24**(2):137–142.

25. Henry MC, Stapleton ER. *EMT. Prehospital Care.* Philadelphia: W.B. Saunders, 1992.

26. Lindner KH, Koster R. Vasopressor drugs during cardiopulmonary resuscitation. *Resuscitation.* 1992;**24**(2):147–154.

27. Oh TE. *Intensive Care Manual.* 3rd ed. Sydney: Butterworths, 1988.

28. Robertson C. The precordial thump and cough techniques in advanced life support. *Resuscitation* 1992;**24**(2):133–136.

29. Robertson C, Holmberg S. Compression techniques and blood flow during cardiopulmonary resuscitation. *Resuscitation* 1992;**24**(2):123–132.

30. Robertson, C, Redmond AD. *The Management of Major Trauma.* Oxford, Oxford University Press, 1991.

31. Safar P, Bircher NG. *Cardiopulmonary Cerebral Resuscitation.* 3rd ed. London: W.B. Saunders (for the World Federation of Societies of Anaesthesiologists Committee on CPR), 1988.

32. Stene JK, Grande CM. *Trauma Anaesthesia.* Baltimore. Williams and Wilkins, 1991.

33. Trunkey DD, Lewis FR. *Current Therapy of Trauma 1984–1985.* Philadelphia: B.C. Decker, 1984.

34. von Planta M, Chamberlain DA. Drug treatment of arrhythmias during cardiopulmonary resuscitation. *Resuscitation* 1992;**24**(2):227–232.

35. Westaby S, ed. *Trauma – Pathogenesis and Treatment.* Oxford: Heinemann, 1989.

36. Woodhouse SP, Lewis-Driver D, Eller H. Catecholamines during cardiopulmonary resuscitation for cardiac arrest. *Resuscitation* 1992;**24**(3):263–272.

INDEX